TABLE OF CONTENTS

Statements of Fact

in Traditional Chinese Medicine

Completely Revised & Expanded

Bob Flaws

Michael Johnston & Timothy Rogers

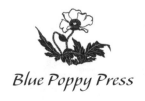

Blue Poppy Press

Published by:
BLUE POPPY PRESS
A Division of Blue Poppy Enterprises, Inc.
5441 Western Ave., Suite 2
BOULDER, CO 80301

First Edition, January, 1994
Second Printing, January, 1996
Third Printing, February, 1998
Second Edition, August, 2001
Fifth Printing, August, 2004
Sixth Printing, July, 2005
Seventh Printing, August, 2006
Third Edition, June, 2008

ISBN 0-936185-52-X

COMP Designation: Original work based on a standard translational terminology
Printed at Sheridan Books, on acid-free paper and soy inks.

10 9 8

Cover & Page Design: Eric J. Brearton

PREFACE

How this book came to be

This is the completely revised and expanded third edition of *Statements of Fact in Traditional Chinese Medicine*. The first edition was published in 1994. It contained a much smaller list of statements along with Chinese characters and Pinyin romanization. The second edition, published in 2001, was a true pocketbook edition, much smaller in format so that it would be easy for students to carry about with them and refer to constantly. (Dare I say it? Like Mao's "little red book".) It contained many more statements than did the first edition. However, it did not contain either Chinese characters or Pinyin romanization and some teachers complained about that. When I was told that *Statements of Fact* would soon be out of stock and needed to be reprinted, I called "time out" and said we needed to do a completely new edition with even more statements but also with the Chinese characters and Pinyin put back in. I had been avoiding this task because it entailed a lot of time-consuming inputting on the computer. However, when it came down to tackling this project, I happened to be teaching a small class on translating modern medical Chinese. When I told this class about this project, two of those students said that they would be willing to do all the inputting from the first edition (the digital files had long been lost) and the collating of the first and second editions. These two students were Michael Johnston, L.Ac. from Ft. Collins, CO, and Timothy Rogers, perennial and peripatetic students of Chinese medicine. So thanks are due to these two stalwarts and their many hours of toggling back and forth between English and Chinese. Their work allowed me to hunt through my library of Chinese medical texts, looking for more statements to include. At the end, all I had to do was to collate all the new statements I had found with Michael and Tim's file. Well, almost all I had to do.

I also have to thank Michael and Tim for one other thing. As they typed in all the statements from the first two editions, they kept wondering exactly what these statements mean in terms of real-life clinical practice. Therefore, they encouraged and finally convinced me to write a commentary for all of the statements appearing in this book based on my reading of the Chinese medical literature and my 30 years practice of this medicine. Although it took a bit of doing, writing this commentary was a very enjoyable and rewarding experience from which I learned a lot. In addition, this version contains a bibliography of all the Chinese texts from which I have culled these statements. I would have liked to identify the actual *locus classicus* of each and every statement contained herein, but that turned out to be simply impossible. Many of my Chinese sources did not give their sources. In any case, what appears here in this edition is a very different book from the first *Statements of Fact*. Hopefully, this edition will be even more useful to students, practitioners, and teachers of Chinese medicine than the first two editions.

All the English language Chinese medical terminology used in this book is based on the work of Nigel Wiseman, Feng Ye, Andrew Ellis, Paul Zmiewski, and others who, over the past 25 years, have created the terminology found in Paradigm Publication's *A Practical Dictionary of Chinese Medicine* (Brookline, MA, 1998). However, although I have used Wiseman *et al.*'s term choices for individual Chinese medical words, I have not necessarily used their translation of whole phrases and sentences. Rather, I have translated them myself using their building blocks. In addition, in the few places where I disagree with Wiseman *et al.*'s term choices, I have tried to footnote these and explain my variances. Words that occur in brackets are words that I have inserted in order to make the terse (and otherwise cryptic) Chinese read intelligibly in English. I have put these words in brackets to help students wanting to learn Chinese to follow more easily from Chinese character to English word in my translation. For the same reason, I have tried to keep the Chinese word order in my translations whenever possible. Further, all of the original Chinese statements are printed in black, while my commentary is printed in blue. Hopefully, this will make differentiation between the Chinese statements themselves and my commentary easier and unambiguous.

What this book is & how to use it

This book is a list of some of the most important statements of fact in Chinese medicine. These are the statements that Chinese doctors (中医生, *zhong yi sheng*) in China use to learn, think and speak about, and, ultimately, practice Chinese medicine. Many of these statements come from the root classics of Chinese medicine—the *Nei Jing (Inner Classic), Nan Jing (Classic of Difficulties), Shang Han Lun (Treatise on Damage [Due to] Cold)*, and the *Jin Gui Yao Lue (Essentials from the Golden Cabinet)*. Others come from famous pre-modern texts written by such pre-eminent authorities as Hua Tuo, Chao Yuan-fang, Sun Si-miao, Zhang Yuan-su, Liu Wan-su, Li Dong-yuan, Zhu Dan-xi, Zhang Jing-yue, Gong Ding-xian, Ye Tian-shi, Tang Zong-hai, and Wang Qing-ren. In my experience as both a student and a teacher, if one memorizes as many of these facts as possible, one will be able to understand and practice Chinese medicine more precisely than those who only have an approximate knowledge of these facts in an imprecise translational terminology.

When I was growing up in the 1950s, we had the politically incorrect but nonetheless entertaining Charlie Chan movies. Those of my generation may remember that, when explaining a perplexing case to his hapless Number One Son, Detective Chan often repeated, "Confucius say" followed by some proverb germane to the situation at hand. To my friends and me, this became an oft-parodied joke. However, Chinese actually do discourse this way. Chinese culture is a culture of consensus, and that consensus is partly based on the frequent repetition of famous quotes and proverbs from authoritative culture heroes. Later, when I was studying Tibetan Buddhism, each class was prefaced by a review of how to be a good student. From the Tibetan Buddhist point of view, there are three mistakes in learning:

1. Memorizing the words but not understanding their meaning
2. Understanding the meaning but not memorizing the words
3. Not remembering the material in the order presented

As a teacher of Chinese medicine in the West having studied Chinese medicine in China, I would say that sometimes Chinese students memorize the words but do not actually understand what they mean. Conversely, it is my experience that Western students understand (at least somewhat) the meaning but rarely remember the actual words. All Chinese doctors in China from Beijing in the north to Tainan in the south, from Shanghai in the east to Chengdu in the west can repeat verbatim a large portion of the statements contained in this book, and these statements act as the armature for pinning and supporting their understanding of this medicine. Their memorization of these statements gives precision and clarity to their remembrance and understanding of Chinese medical theory.

Further, when reading the Chinese medical literature in Chinese, it is clear that Chinese doctors think and solve clinical problems by arranging these various statements in logical syllogisms. In my experience, Chinese doctors tend to think in a highly logical and systematic way, with the statements contained herein comprising the fundamental propositions with which they reason. For those unfamiliar with the concept of a syllogism, the commonly used example of a simple categorical deductive syllogism goes like this:

Proposition A: All humans are mortal.
Proposition B: Socrates is a human.

Deduction: Therefore, Socrates will die.

In this case, two statements of fact are arranged in such a way that they produce a new piece of knowledge, a new fact, and this is exactly how Chinese doctors think, speak, and write and develop their understanding and practice of this medicine.[1] The following is an example of a multi-proposition or multi-premise Chinese medical syllogism constructed from statements found within this book.

Premise A: The spleen governs the movement and
    transformation of water fluids.
Premise B: If water fluids collect (*i.e.*, stop moving), they
    transform into dampness.
Premise C: If dampness endures, it congeals into phlegm.
    Deduction (or summation): Therefore, the spleen is the
    source of phlegm engenderment.

To some extent, the more of these statements of fact one memorizes, the more Chinese medical problems you will be able to solve. I like to compare the memorization of these statements to the uploading of a computer program where these statements are the operating code. Once the program is up-loaded correctly and completely, one can solve all sorts of problems with that program. However, if the software is faulty or incomplete, then the program simply does not work.

As for how to use this book, it is not a stand-alone basic theory text. However, its use can greatly help in learning the theory in such basic texts. Therefore, I recommend that students study this book along with whatever basic theory text their school has chosen. Then, along with understanding the theory contained in that text, they should try to memorize as many of the corresponding statements of fact as possible. That way, one will have remembered the words *and* understood their meaning. Secondly, I recommend teachers of Chinese medicine use as

---

[1] In point of fact, categorical deductive syllogisms do not actually create new facts. Rather, they reveal facts that may have been only implied but not previously explicitly stated.

many of these statements as possible in their classes, repeating them over and over again so that their students become used to hearing them. In my experience, if one really wants to master this system of medicine, one should pickle themselves in these famous statements of fact. And third, I recommend practitioners use these statements when conversing with each other. In my opinion, one of the problems with the practice of Chinese medicine in the West is that, due to not having a standard translational terminology or a standard fund of essential knowledge, we are often confused when talking to each other. Are we talking about the same things? Are our conversations and our logic true to Chinese medicine as created and practiced in the land of its origin? By using these statements as the irreducible facts of our art, we can converse and, indeed, debate with some commonly agreed knowledge as our basis. Therefore, I do not just recommend students and practitioners read this book. Rather, I hope they will ponder, if not meditate on, these statements and commit as many of them to memory as possible.

Good luck and best wishes.

Bob Flaws
Boulder, CO

February 14, 2007

CHINESE MEDICINE BASIC THEORY
(中医基础理论, *zhong yi ji chu li lun*)

Perhaps the single most important word in Chinese medicine is
"correspondence" (应, *ying*). This means that two entities which
might otherwise seem unrelated are linked in a bidirectional
manner so that they respond to each other. This means that what
affects one member of the pair may and commonly does affect
the other member and *vice versa*. It is this concept of correspondence which makes Chinese medicine holistic both in terms of
the body and the world at large and the body and its individual
parts. Within Chinese medicine, the two main systems of
correspondence are yin-yang and the five phases. Although these
arose as separate philosophical schools, they eventually became
blended. For over two millennia, Chinese medicine has been a
medicine of systematic correspondence. However, before
looking at the statements of fact pertaining to yin and yang and
the five phases, there are some general, broader statements about
the creation of the phenomenal world and humanity's place
within that world.

Below heaven, the tens of thousands of things are engendered
from something, and something is engendered from nothing.
(天下万物生于有，有生于无。 *Tian xia wan wu sheng yu you,
you sheng yu wu.*)
> This statement by Lao-zi states that the phenomenal universe is
> created out of nothing. This nothing is also called absolute nothing-
> ness (无极, *wu ji*) or the *dao* (道).

Heaven [and] earth are the up [and] down of the tens of thousands of things. (天地者，万物之上下也。 *Tian di zhe, wan wu zhi shang xia ye.*)

  This statement implies that it is heaven above and earth below that create the tens of thousands of things.

Heaven, earth, and humanity are the three abilities. (三才者，天地人也。 *San cai zhe, tian di ren ye.*)

  Within the phenomenal universe, the three main things that make other things happen are heaven, earth, and humanity. In other words, once created, humans become an equally potent agency for change in the world.

Heaven, earth, [and] humanity are mutually interconnected as one. (天地人相统一. *Tian di ren xiang tong yi.*)

  This means that whatever happens in the heavens affects the earth and vice versa. It also means that whatever happens in the heavens or on the earth affects humans, including the state of our health. However, likewise, human activities can also affect the state of the heavens and/or earth. Therefore, all three are mutually interdependent.

Humans are engendered by the qi of heaven [and] earth. (人以天地之气生。 *Ren yi tian di zhi qi sheng.*)

  Here, heaven and earth stand for yang and yin respectively, while qi is that which engenders and activates us humans.

Heaven feeds humans the five qi; earth feeds humans the five flavors. (天食人以五气，地食人以五味。 *Tian shi ren yi wu qi, di shi ren yi wu wei.*)

  The five qi of heaven are the five seasons or, more specifically, the weather of the five seasons—spring, summer, long summer, fall, and winter. These five seasons correspond to the five phases—wood, fire, earth, metal, and water. Therefore, one can also say that the five qi of heaven are the five phases. The five flavors are the five flavors of food—sweet, sour, acrid, bitter, and salty. These five flavors come from the earth since all food comes either directly or indirectly from the earth.

Upbearing [and] downbearing are the interaction of the qi of heaven [and] earth. (升降者，天地之气交也。 *Sheng jiang zhe, tian di zhi qi jiao ye.*)

> In this statement, 交 (*jiao*) means to interact but, more literally, means to join as in intercourse where one thing penetrates and joins with another. In this case, the qi of heaven should downbear and join with earth, while the qi of earth should upbear and join with heaven.

Heaven's qi ascends [and] upbears, earth's qi descends [and] downbears. (天气上升，地气下降也。 *Tian qi shang sheng, di qi xia jiang ye.*)

Heaven is light, clear, and floats upward. Earth is heavy, turbid, and descends and congeals. (天者，轻清而上浮也。地者，重浊而下凝也。 *Tian zhe, qing qing er shang fu ye. Di zhe, chong zhuo er xia ning ye.*)

> The characteristics of heaven and earth are essentially the characteristics of yang and yin respectively. Here, the characteristics of heaven and earth are juxtaposed but still described individually. It is only when describing the inter-relationship of heaven and earth should heaven's qi descend and earth's qi ascend.

Because heaven [and] humanity mutually affect [and] mutually correspond, heaven's loss of normalcy leads to disaster, [while] humans' loss of normalcy leads to disease. [Nevertheless,] disaster can be prevented, and disease can be treated. Both are connected by one qi. (因而天人相感相应，天失常则灾，人失常则病，灾可防而病可治，皆统一于气。 *Yin er tian ren xiang gan xiang ying, tian shi chang ze zai, ren shi chang ze bing, zai ke fang er bing ke zhi, jie tong yi yu qi.*)

> According to this statement, heaven and humanity partake of a single qi which unites the two. When heaven loses its normalcy, this results in natural disasters. When humans lose their normalcy, this results in disease.

The engenderment of things is called their transformation; the

end of things is called their change. (物生谓之化，物极谓之
变。 *Wu sheng wei zhi hua, wu ji wei zhi bian.*)

This statement is basically a clarification of semantics. The word
"transformation" implies something being engendered or created,
while the word "change" implies a change resulting in the end or
death of something.

Humans' life is 100 years and [then we] die. (人之寿百岁而
死。 *Ren zhi shou bai sui er si.*)

According to this statement from the *Ling Shu (Spiritual Axis)*, the
natural human lifespan is 100 years.

YIN-YANG THEORY
(阴阳学说, *yin yang xue shuo*)

Originally, yin-yang theory was one of the ancient schools of philosophy in China. However, by the Warring States period (476-221 BCE), this theory had been applied to Chinese medicine. According to this theory, everything in the phenomenal universe has a yin and yang aspect. These two apsects are mutually opposed but also mutually united, the two faces of a single thing. It is due to these two fundamental aspects or characteristics of phenomenal reality that things change and transform.

In general, yang represents activity, function, warmth, and movement, while yin represents matter, form, cold, and stillness.

Yin & Yang
(阴阳, *yin yang*)

Absolute nothingness engenders the supreme ultimate; the supreme ultimate engenders the two yi; the two yi engender the four images; and the four images engender the eight trigrams. (无极生太极，太极生两仪，两仪生四象，四象生八卦。*Wu ji sheng tai ji, tai ji sheng liang yi, liang yi sheng si xiang, si xiang sheng ba gua.*)

> This statement explains how the *tai ji*, the indivisible unity of all things arises out of absolute nothingness. Then the *tai ji* engenders the two appearances. These are yin and yang. Yin and yang then go

on to multiply into four, the four images, and four is multiplied into eight, the eight trigrams of the *Yi Jing (Classic of Changes).*

One yin [and] one yang are called the dao. (一阴一阳谓之道。 *Yi yin yi yang wei zhi dao.*)

The dao is made from one yin [and] one yang. (一阴一阳为之 道。 *Yi yin yi yang wei zhi dao.*)

Yin [and] yang are the dao of heaven [and] earth. (阴阳者，天 地之道也。 *Yin yang zhe, tian di zhi dao ye.*)

[When] yin [and] yang [are] unfathomable, [this is what] is called spirit. (阴阳不测谓之神。 *Yin yang bu ce wei zhi shen.*)
"When yin and yang are unfathomable" refers to the state before the seeming separation of yin and yang.

Yin and yang are one divided into two. (阴阳者，一分为二 也。 *Yin yang zhe, yi fen wei er ye.*)

One divided makes two. (一分为二。 *Yi fen wei er.*)
The separation or dualism of yin and yang are only apparent due to the limitations of the human mind.

Both yin [and] yang have a name but no form. (且夫阴阳者, 有 名而无形。 *Qie fu yin yang zhe, you ming er wu xing.*)
In other words, yin and yang are only abstract concepts.

The essence of yang is the sun. (阳之精者为日。 *Yang zhi jing zhe wei ri.*)

The essence of yin is the moon. (阴之精者为月。 *Yin zhi jing zhe wei yue.*)
Within our world, the essence of yang is the sun and the essence of yin is the moon. In fact, 太阳 (*tai yang*) is another name for the sun.

The root of life [is] rooted in yin [and] yang. (生之本，本于阴
阳。 *Sheng zhi ben, ben yu yin yang.*)

All life is rooted in yin and yang. In other words, yin and yang are
concepts which can be applied to all life. There is no living thing
which cannot be described in terms of yin and yang or no living
process that cannot be described in terms of yin and yang.

The accumulation of yang makes heaven; the accumulation of
yin makes earth. (积阳为天，积阴为地。 *Ji yang wei tian, ji yin
wei di.*)

This statement makes clear that heaven is yang and earth is yin.

[Once] a human is born [and] has form, [they] cannot be
separated from yin [and] yang. (人生有形，不离阴阳 *Ren
sheng you xing, bu li yin yang.*)

This statement makes it clear that yin and yang also pertain to the
human body and its life activities just as they do to all the rest of
phenomenal existence. Therefore, all the following statements
about yin and yang have their medical implications and applications.

The word "engender" (生, *sheng,* which also means "life," "living,"
"to be born," and "to grow") is routinely associated below with
yang function, while the word "form" (形, *xing*) always implies yin
substance or material basis.

Humanity's engenderment [or life] has hard and soft, short and
long, yin and yang. (人之生也，有刚有柔，有短有长，有阴
有阳。 *Ren zhi sheng ye, you gang you rou, you duan you chang,
you yin you yang.*)

This statement further substantiates that human life corresponds to
yin and yang. Therefore, the concepts of yin and yang can be used
in medicine.

Yang is rooted in yin; yin is rooted in yang; yin and yang are
mutually rooted. (阳根于阴，阴根于阳，阴阳互根 *Yang gen
yu yin, yin gen yu yang, yin yang hu gen.*)

This means that yin and yang cannot be separated. Although they
are spoken of as two, they are the two aspects of a single unitary
reality.

Yin is engendered by yang. (阴生于阳 *Yin sheng yu yang.*)
It is yang's active function which engenders yin.

Yang is engendered from yin. (阳生于阴 *Yang sheng yu yin.*)
Yin is the fuel or substance from which yang is engendered and
transformed.

Yin obtaining yang's assistance leads to the source spring [being]
inexhaustible. (阴得阳助则泉源不竭。 *Yin de yang zhu ze quan
yuan bu jie.*)

Yang obtaining yin's assistance leads to upbearing [and]
transformation being limitless. (阳得阴助则升化无穷。 *Yang de
yin zhu ze sheng hua wu qiong.*)
As long as there is sufficient fuel, yang's function is limitless.

Yin and yang may change and transform [into each other].
(阴阳转化 *Yin yang zhuan hua.*)
These statements all state that yin and yang are mutually engendering. It takes yin to make yang and yang to make yin and neither is
primary.

Heaven has yin [and] yang, [and] earth also has yin [and] yang.
(天有阴阳，地亦有阴阳。 *Tian you yin yang, di yi you yin yang.*)
If heaven is yang, this statement means that there is both yin and
yang within yang. If earth is yin, then there is likewise yin and yang
within yin.

[There is] yang within yang [and] yin within yang. (阳中之阳，
阳中之阴 *Yang zhong zhi yang; yang zhong zhi yin.*)

[There is] yin within yin [and] yang within yin. (阴中之阴， 阴
中之阳 *Yin zhong zhi yin; yin zhong zhi yang.*)
Nothing is wholly yin or wholly yang. As the following ancient
Chinese chart shows, yin and yang may be subdivided infinitely into
yin within yang and yang within yin.

Yin and yang disperse and grow [*i.e,.* wax and wane].
(阴阳消长 *Yin yang xiao zhang.*)

The relative proportions of yin and yang are constantly changing and never static. Typically, if one waxes, the other wanes.

Double yang necessarily [transforms into] yin. (重阳必阴 *Chong yang bi yin.*)

When yang reaches its apogee or extreme (至, *zhi*), it transforms into yin.

Double yin necessarily [transforms into] yang. (重阴必阳 *Chong yin bi yang.*)

When yin reaches its apogee or extreme, it transforms into yang. In other words, when either yin or yang grow to their extreme, they spontaneously transform into their opposite.

Yin and yang are sympathetic. (阴阳交感 *Yin yang jiao gan.*)

When either yin or yang changes, this likewise affects its opposite.

Yin and yang may recur [and recuperate]. (阴阳胜复 *Yin yang sheng fu.*)

This means that temporary prevalence of yin or yang occur and eventually right themselves in a ceaseless cycle.

[When] yang is exuberant, yin is repelled. (阳盛格阴 *Yang sheng ge yin.*)

[When] yang is exuberant, yin is damaged. (阳盛阴伤 *Yang sheng yin shang.*)

These two statements both explain that the waxing of yang commonly leads to the waning of yin.

Yin exuberance repels yang. (阴盛格阳 *Yin sheng ge yang.*)

[When] yin is exuberant, yang is debilitated. (阴盛阳衰 *Yin sheng yang shuai.*)

Yin exuberance leads to yang [becoming] diseased. (阴盛则阳病 *Yin sheng ze yang bing.*)

These three statements, on the other hand, explain that the waxing of yin commonly leads to the waning of yang.

Detriment of yin affects [or reaches] yang. (阴损及阳 *Yin sun ji yang*.)

Detriment of yang affects [or reaches] yin. (阳损及阴 *Yang sun ji yin*.)
However, because yin and yang are mutually rooted, excessive damage to one will also eventually lead to damage to the other.

Yin and yang may become spontaneously harmonious. (阴阳自和 *Yin yang zi he*.)
It is also possible for yin and yang to spontaneously restore their dynamic balance.

[When] yang engenders, yin lengthens [or grows]. (阳生阴长 *Yang sheng yin zhang*.)
When in harmonious relationship, yin and yang mutually benefit each other. In particular, it is the engendering function of yang which leads to the growth of yin.

Without yang, yin cannot transform; without yin, yang cannot engender. (无阳则阴无以化，无阴则阳无以生 *Wu yang ze yin wu yi hua, wu yin ze yang wu yi sheng*.)
Yin and yang are like flame and fuel in an engine. Yang transforms yin which engenders more yang activity. However, the function of yang can then also manufacture more fuel if given the raw materials to work on. In general, within the human body, yin should be thought of as matter, form, and fuel, and yang should be thought of as function.

[When] yin is level [*i.e.,* calm], yang is secret [*i.e.,* unobtrusive, sound]. (阴平阳秘 *Yin ping yang mi*.)

[If] yin is level [or calm and] yang is secreted, the essence spirit [or psyche] is therefore in order [or at peace]. (阴平阳秘，精神乃治。 *Yin ping yang mi, jing shen nai zhi*.)
These two statements exhibit the Chinese preference for harmony and calmness as opposed to rebelliousness and chaos. In particular, yang should not be too excessive or there will be too much stirring and hyperactivity. The latter statement goes on to explain how, if

yin and yang are healthy, the human psyche is also healthy and in order.

[When] yang is killed, yin is stored. (阳杀阴藏 *Yang sha yin cang.*)

If yang is "killed" or prevented from being hyperactive or having a surplus, then yin can be stored.

Yang commonly has a surplus; yin is commonly insufficient. (阳常有余，阴常不足 *Yang chang you yu, yin chang bu zu.*)

However, within the human body, yin and yang are not equal. If they were, this would produce a static balance with lack of any movement or change. Therefore, yang is slightly more abundant than yin. The downside of this is that there is also a tendency for yang to become hyperactive.

Yin may fail to embrace yang. (阴不包阳 *Yin bu bao yang.*)

If yin fails to restrain yang, then yang stirs and becomes hyperactive.

[When] yang is strong and is not able to be consolidated, yin qi expires. (阳强不能密，阴气乃绝 *Yang qiang bu neng mi, yin qi nai jue.*)

If yang becomes too strong and exuberant, too hyperactive, it consumes and damages yin which eventually becomes exhausted and expires.

[When] yin and yang separate, essence and qi expire. (阴阳离决，精气乃绝 *Yin yang li jue, jing qi nai jue.*)

If the imbalance between yin and yang becomes too severe, yin and yang may come apart. When that happens in a human being, the person dies.

Yang transforms the qi; yin produces the form. (阳化气，阴成形 *Yang hua qi, yin cheng xing.*)

This statement explains the fundamental functions of yin and yang within the human body.

Yin [and] yang are the blood [and] qi of men [and] women. (阴阳者，血气之男女也。 *Yin yang zhe, xue qi zhi nan nu ye.*)

Within the body, yin and yang are functionally the blood and qi in both men and women.

The six bowels are yang; the five viscera are yin. (六腑为阳，五脏为阴 *Liu fu wei yang, wu zang wei yin.*)
> According to yin-yang theory, the six bowels are yang compared to the five viscera which are yin.

[If] yin exists internally, yang [has a place] to abide. (阴在内，阳之守也。*Yin zai nei, yang zhi shou ye.*)
> Yin existing internally provides an anchor for yang externally so that it does not float up and away from the body.

[If] yang qi is effulgent, the five viscera receive boons. (阳气旺则五脏受荫 *Yang qi wang ze wu zang shou yin.*)
> The five viscera depend on yang qi to do their function, and their function is to store essence or "boons."

Yang is able to transform qi; qi is able to transform water. (阳能化气，气能化水 *Yang neng hua qi, qi neng hua shui.*)
> The idea here is that yang precedes qi. Then qi is able to transform water which is yin.

Clear yang exits from the upper portals; turbid yin exits from the lower portals. (清阳出上窍，浊阴出下窍 *Qing yang chu shang qiao, zhuo yin chu xia qiao.*)

Clear yang is emitted from the interstices; turbid yin penetrates the five viscera. (清阳发凑理，浊阴走五脏 *Qing yang fa cou li, zhuo yin zou wu zang.*)

Clear yang is replete in the four extremities; turbid yin returns to the six bowels. (清阳实四肢，浊阴归六腑 *Qing yang shi si zhi, zhuo yin gui liu fu.*)
> Here, clear yang refers to the clear yang qi derived from the clearest part of the finest essence of food and drink. The turbid yin is the turbid residue of the process of digestion. Ultimately, the dregs of this turbid residue are excreted from the body as urine and feces.

[In] the spring [and] summer, the yang qi [is] a lot [and] the yin qi [is] less. (春夏则阳气多而阴气少。 *Chun xia ze yang qi duo er yin qi shao.*)

[In] the fall [and] winter, the yin qi [is] exuberant [and] the yang qi is debilitated. (秋冬则阴气盛而阳气衰。 *Qiu dong ze yin qi sheng er yang qi shuai.*)

These last two statements explain the relative proportions of yin and yang in the various seasons.

Above is yang, below is yin. (上为阳，下为阴。 *Shang wei yang, xia wei yin.*)

In other words, the upper body is relatively yang and the lower body is relatively yin.

Qi is yang, blood is yin. (气为阳，血为阴。 *Qi wei yang, xue wei yin.*)

When qi and blood are compared together, qi is relatively yang and blood is relatively yin.

Yin exists internally; yang exists externally. (阴在内，阳在外。 *Yin zai nei, yang zai wai.*)

The exterior is yang, the interior is yin. (表为阳，里为阴。 *Biao wei yang, li wei yin.*)

When the interior of the body is compared to the exterior of the body, the interior is relatively yin while the exterior is relatively yang.

The upper back is yang, [and] the lungs are yin within yang. (背为阳，阳中之阴肺也。 *Bei wei yang, yang zhong zhi yin fei ye.*)

The upper back as a whole is yang, but the lungs within the upper back are relatively yin within yang.

A liking for brightness is yang, a desire for dark is yin. (喜明者为阳，欲暗者为阴。 *Xi ming zhe wei yang, yu an zhe wei yin.*)
Yin existing internally is observed via yang [externally]. (阴在内阳之守也 *Yin zai nei yang zhi shou ye.*)

Yang existing externally represents yin [internally]. (阳在外阴
之使也 *Yang zai wai yin zhi shi ye.*)

> Both these statements explain that the nature of yin internally
> manifests signs or symptoms affecting yang one way or another
> externally.

[At] 40 years [of age], yin qi is automatically half. (年四十，而
阴气自半也。*Nian si shi, er yin qi si ban ye.*)

> According to the *Nei Jing (Inner Classic)*, by 40 years of age, a
> person has transformed and consumed approximately half their
> former heaven yin through the various activities of living.

Yang vacuity [is] easy to treat; yin vacuity [is] difficult to
regulate. (阳虚易治，阴虚难调。*Yang xu yi zhi, yin xu nan
tiao.*)

> In practice, yang vacuity responds relatively quickly to treatment
> such as with warming and invigorating medicinals or with
> moxibustion. However, yin is not so easy to supplement. Yin is
> substance and must be engendered and grow back over time.

FIVE PHASES
(五行, *wu xing*)

Five Phase Theory
(五行学说 *wu xing xue shuo*)

Like yin yang theory above, five phase theory was also one of the ancient schools of philosophy in China. Similarly, by the Warring States period (476-221 BCE), it too had been applied to Chinese medicine. According to this theory, all of phenomenal reality corresponds to the properties of the five phases, *i.e.,* wood, fire, earth, metal, and water, and these properties are mutually interdependent, mutually engendering, and mutually restraining. This theory allows for a larger, more complex mechanism of change and transformation in nature.

Heaven has five movements [or phases]. (天有五行。 *Tian you wu xing.*)
   The early understanding of the five phases seems to have been based on observation of the four or five seasons.

Spring [is] birth, summer [is] growth, fall [is] harvesting, winter [is] storage. These are the normal qi, [and] humans also correspond [to them]. (春生，夏长，秋收，冬藏，是气之常也，人亦应之。 *Chun sheng, xia chang, qiu shou, dong cang, shi qi zhi zhang ye, ren yi ying zhi.*)
   The wood phase corresponds to spring and, therefore, birth. The

fire phase corresponds to summer and, therefore, growth. The metal phase corresponds to fall and, therefore, harvesting, while the water phase corresponds to winter and, therefore, storage.

The five phases are, metal, wood, water, fire, [and] earth. (五行者，金木水火土也。 *Wu xing zhe, jin mu shui huo tu ye*.)

Earth is the center of the five phases. (土五行之中也。 *Tu wu xing zhi zhong ye*.)
  Placing earth in the center this way helps explain why only the four seasons are discussed above.

The five movements govern disease—wood, fire, earth, metal, [and] water. [Their] normal movement leads to everything being still. [Their] counterflow leads to change [and] chaos. (五运主病木火土金水顺则皆静，逆则变乱。 *Wu yun zhu bing mu huo tu jin shui shun ze jie jing, ni ze bian luan*.)
  The five phases are sometimes also called the five movements. When these five flow normally, everything is still and tranquil. However, if they counterflow or flow abnormally, this then results in pathological changes and chaos.

Mutual Engenderment
(相生, *xiang sheng*)

Mutual engenderment means that, when the five phases are plotted on the circumference of a circle, each phase moving in a clockwise manner engenders the succeeding phase. Thus wood engenders fire, fire engenders earth, earth engenders metal, metal engenders water, and water engenders wood.

The five phases mutually engender. (五行相生。 *Wu xing xiang sheng*.)
  The five phases mutually engender one another.

Mutual restraint
(相克, *xiang ke*)

Mutual restraint means that each phase controls or restrains the next plus one phase after it. Thus wood restrains earth, earth restrains water, water restrains fire, fire restrains metal, and metal restrains wood.

The five phases mutually restrain. (五行相克。 *Wu xing xiang ke.*)
  The five phases mutually restrain one another.

The five phases [may] mutually overwhelm. (五行相乘。 *Wu xing xiang cheng.*)
  Mutual overwhelming means that a phase not only restrains another phase but actually attacks and overwhelms it to that second phase's detriment.

The five phases [may] mutually rebel. (五行相侮。 *Wu xing xiang wu.*)
  Mutual rebellion is when a phase rebels back upon and damages the phase that would normally restrain it according to the control cycle.

The five phases control [and] transform [one another]. (五行制化。 *Wu xing zhi hua.*)
  Thus do the five phases control and transform into one another.

The five phases mother [and] child mutually reach [or affect one another]. (五行母子相及。 *Wu xing mu zi xiang ji.*)
  According to the engenderment cycle, each of the five phases is the mother to its succeeding phase, its child, and these mothers and their children can affect each other.

Disease of the mother may affect the child. (母病及子 *Mu bing ji zi.*)
  This describes the process whereby the disease of a mother organ eventually causes disease in a child organ according to the engenderment cycle.

Disease of the child [may] reach the mother. (子病及母 *Zi bing ji mu.*)

The child [may] steal the mother's qi. (子盗母气 *Zi dao mu qi.*)
This describes the process whereby the disease of a child organ is transmitted "backwards" to a mother organ according to the engenderment cycle. In particular, the second statement implies that vacuity[1] of the child may result in vacuity of the mother.

Wood
(木, *mu*)

Wood is the beginning of the five phases; water is the end of the five phases. (木，五行之始也；水，五行之终也。*Mu, wu xing zhi shi ye; shui, wu xing zhi zhong ye.*)
Wood corresponds to birth and, therefore, the beginning or birth of things. Water corresponds to storage and stillness and, therefore, the end of things. When listing the five phases, one usually begins with wood and follows the engenderment cycle ending with water.

Wood likes orderly reaching. (木喜条达 *Mu xi tiao da.*)
In terms of Chinese medicine, this means that the liver qi likes or has a predilection to spread and flow freely without hindrance or blockage.

Wood depression not spreading leads to the causation [and] engenderment of hundreds of diseases. (木郁不达，则百病由生。*Mu yu bu da, ze bai bing you sheng.*)
Here, wood depression is another way of saying liver depression qi stagnation (肝郁气滞, *gan yu qi zhi*), and liver depression qi

---

[1] 虚 (*xu*) is translated as "vacuity" by Wiseman *et al.* Many English-speakers use the word "deficiency." In fact, the simplest English translation of this word would be "emptiness." However, the more common Chinese word for emptiness, 空 (*kong*) is also used in Chinese medicine. Therefore, Wiseman *et al.* have resorted to a less frequently used word for emptiness, vacuity.

stagnation causes or complicates many, many other conditions. In clinical practice, it is rare to see a chronic, enduring condition in which there is not an element of liver depression. According to Yan De-xin, liver depression plays a part in all chronic, enduring diseases whether or not liver depression was the initial, precipitating cause of the disease.

Wood is called the bending [and] straightening. (木曰曲直 *Mu yue qu zhi.*)

In terms of medicine, this suggests that diseases affecting the flexion and extension of the joints often involve the sinews which correspond to liver-wood. In particular, if the sinews are inadequately nourished by blood, they become dry and may contract, thus preventing their extension or "straightening."

Depression of wood transforms [into] fire. (木郁化火 *Mu yu hua huo.*)

If the liver become depressed and its qi stagnant, because the qi is yang and, therefore, inherently warm in nature, this depression may transform into evil heat or, if extreme, fire. This is called depressive or transformative heat or fire.

Wood fire torments metal. (木火刑金 *Mu huo xing jin.*)

Depressive liver heat may cause lung disease. All heat by nature tends to float upward, and the lungs are the "florid canopy" covering all the other viscera and bowels. Therefore, depressive heat often accumulates in the lungs, disturbing the lungs' depuration and downbearing or diffusing and downbearing. When the lungs cannot diffuse and downbear, this gives rise to coughing and the accumulation of phlegm.

Wood [may] check earth. (木克土 *Mu ke tu.*)

Wood effulgence overwhelms earth. (木旺乘土。 *Mu wang cheng tu.*)

Liver depression qi stagnation is a wood repletion pattern. In this case, the liver qi may easily and commonly does counterflow horizontally to assail the spleen and/or stomach. In this case, the spleen typically becomes vacuous and the stomach becomes disharmonious and potentially hot.

Depression of wood transforms [into] wind. (木郁化风 *Mu yu hua feng.*)

Liver depression qi stagnation may give rise to depressive heat. If this heat further transforms into fire effulgence or yang hyperactivity, it may give rise to internal stirring of liver wind. Internal strirring of liver wind may also be due to depressive heat damaging and consuming yin and blood. In that case, yin may fail to control yang and liver wind may stir internally.

Wood is able to course earth. (木能疏土。 *Mu neng shu tu.*)

The liver corresponds to the wood phase. It is the liver qi's governance over coursing and discharge which keeps the qi mechanism freely flowing and uninhibited. Because the qi mechanism describes the integrated upbearing of the spleen and downbearing of the stomach and the spleen and stomach correspond to the earth phase, wood is able to course earth.

Fire
(火, *huo*)

Fire's nature is to flame upward. (火性上炎 *Huo xing shang yan.*)

All heat by nature tends to float or flare upward in the body no matter how it was originally engendered. Therefore, internally engendered heat of all types tends to eventually accumulate in the heart and/or lungs.

Fire is called the flaming [and] ascending. (火曰炎上。 *Huo yue yan shang.*)

This statement reiterates the preceding statement that fire's nature is to flame upward.

Exuberant fire torments metal. (火盛刑金 *Huo sheng xing jin.*)

In clinical practice, this mostly describes the process of liver fire resulting in or aggravating lung disease.

Fire [may] not engender earth. (火不生土 *Huo bu sheng tu.*)

Heart vacuity may give rise to spleen vacuity.

[For] fire depression, effuse [it]. (火郁发之。 *Huo yu fa zhi.*)
This means that depressive heat or fire transformed from
depressive heat should be effused or out-thrust from the body
using acrid, windy-natured medicinals or other such treatment
methods to effuse and out-thrust.

Earth
(土, *tu*)

Earth engenders the tens of thousands of things. (土生万物　*Tu
sheng wan wu.*)
In medicine, the spleen and stomach correspond to the earth phase
and are the latter heaven root of the engenderment and
transformation of the qi and blood. Because the qi and blood
construct and nourish all the other organs and tissues of the body,
the spleen and stomach are likened to the earth from which all
plants and animals spring.

Earth is the mother of [all] things. The heart, liver, lungs, and
kidneys [are] like [her] four children. [If] the child is vacuous,
[one] can rely on the generosity of the mother qi. (土为物母，
心肝肺肾若四子焉，子虚尚可仰给母气。 *Tu wei wu mu, xin
gan fei shen ruo si zi yan, zi shu shang ke yang ji mu qi.*)
This statement is a corollary of the above. Earth or the spleen is the
mother of all the other viscera in the body since it is the spleen
which is the root or source of the qi and blood which construct
and nourish all the other viscera.

Earth plus metal, wood, water, [and] fire produce the hundreds
of things. (以土与金木水火杂以成百物。 *Yi tu yu jin mu shui
huo za yi cheng bai wu.*)

Earth is the mother of the tens of thousands of things. (土为万物
之母。 *Tu wei wan wu zhi mu.*)

The tens of thousands of things are born within the earth; the tens
of thousands of things are extinguished within the earth. (万物土
中生，万物土中灭。 *Wan wu tu zhong sheng, wan wu tu zhong mie.*)

All these statements reiterate the central primacy of the earth.

Earth likes warmth [and] dryness. (土喜温燥 *Tu xi wen zao.*)

In terms of medicine, the function of the spleen is nothing other than the function of its yang qi, and yang qi is inherently warm. Further, both internally engendered and externally contracted damp evils may damage and encumber the function of the spleen. Clinically, this means that eating or administering too many cool and cold foods or medicinals can damage the spleen as can overeating too many foods which strongly engender fluids. If too many foods which strongly engender fluids are eaten, these may engender dampness which then damages and encumbers the spleen.

Earth [may] not control water. (土不制水 *Tu bu zhi shui.*)

This statement relates to the spleen and stomach's role in the movement and transformation of water fluids in the body. If, due to qi vacuity, the spleen fails to move and transform water fluids adequately, these may collect and then spill over in the body causing various damp accumulations and water swellings within the body. It is also possible that, due to heat and consequent hyperactivity, the stomach may downbear too many fluids to the kidneys and bladder, thus resulting in polyuria.

Earth [may] not engender metal. (土不生金 *Tu bu sheng jin.*)

In clinical practice, spleen qi vacuity may give rise to lung qi vacuity. This may then manifest as such signs and symptoms as a faint, weak voice, disinclination or laziness to speak, spontaneous perspiration, and/or easy contraction of external evils.

Vacuous earth [may] be overwhelmed by wood. (土虚木乘。 *Tu xu mu cheng.*)

If earth is vacuous, it is easy for wood to overwhelm it. Clinically, this means that spleen vacuity allows the liver to become effulgent and overwhelm the spleen.

[If] earth [is] vacuous, water [may] rebel. (土虚水侮。 *Tu xu shui wu.*)

This means that if earth is vacuous, water may rebel against it. In clinical practice, this implies spleen vacuity may give rise to dampness.

Depressed earth [is treated by] despoiling. (土郁夺之 *Tu yu duo zhi.*)

> Essentially, despoiling here refers to draining the middle burner. For instance, depressed dampness may either be dried or seeped and depressed food may be dispersed and abducted.

Earth is called the sowing [and] hoarding. (土曰稼穑 *Tu yue jia se.*)

> Just as food crops are sown and then ripen due to the agency of the earth, so the spleen and stomach, the earth organs, are the root and source of the qi, blood, fluids, and latter heaven essence in the body.

Earth has high [and] low; qi has warm [and] cool. High [altitude's] qi [is] cold; low [altitude's] qi [is] hot. (地有高下，气有温凉，高者气寒，低者气热。 *Di you gao xia, qi you wen liang, gao zhe qi han, di zhe qi re.*)

> Here earth (地, *di*) refers more to the physical earth than the abstract earth (土, *tu*) phase. As such, this statement is merely a reflection of the fact that early Chinese well understood that the temperature of the air decreases typically as one gains altitude.

Metal
(金, *jin*)

Metal is called the bellows. (金曰从革。 *Jin yue cong ge.*)

> Here metal refers to the lungs which are the bellows of the body, driving air in and out via respiration.

Replete metal fails to sound. (金实不鸣 *Jin shi by ming.*)

> Replete metal refers to evils lodged in the lungs, the metal viscus. In that case, the lung qi does not diffuse and downbear correctly. One of the symptoms of this lack of adequate diffusion and down-bearing is hoarseness and indistinct speech.

Metal [and] water engender each other. (金水相生 *Jin shui xiang sheng.*)

Normally, metal engenders water according to the engenderment cycle. However, in clinical practice, lung qi and/or yin vacuity may give rise to kidney qi and/or yin vacuity and vice versa.

Depressed metal [is treated by] draining. (金郁泻之 *Jin yu xie zhi.*)

Depressed metal refers to evils lodged in the lungs. Wind evils need to be drained by coursing and out-thrusting, while phlegm rheum needs to be drained by transforming and expelling. All these treatment methods fall under the broad category of draining in Chinese medicine.

Metal qi depurates [and] downbears. (金气肃降 *Jin qi su jiang.*)

This refers to the lung qi's function of spreading the qi and water fluids "downward" throughout the body.

Metal [is] cold; water [is] frigid. (金寒水冷 *Jin han shui leng.*)

Comparatively, the lungs are yang within yin, while the kidneys are yin within yin.

Water
(水, *shui*)

Water's nature is to flow downward. (水性流下 *Shui xing liu xia.*)

Just as heat's nature is to flow upward, water's nature in the body is to flow downward. Unless the spleen qi actively upbears the clear part of water fluids, these will tend to fall downward, moving from the middle to the lower burner. This pathological downward movement of water fluids in the body manifests as such signs and symptoms as dropsy (*i.e.,* edema of the lower extremities), polyuria, and abnormal vaginal discharge. In addition, the main avenue for discharge of excess fluids from the body is for it to move downward via the yin tract for discharge from the kidneys and bladder as urine.

Water is called the moistening [and] descending. (水曰润下。 *Shui yue run xia.*)

This statement reiterates water's nature as being moistening and descending.

Water [may] not moisten wood. (水不涵木 *Shui bu han mu.*)
Just as with all other organs and tissues in the body, for the liver to
function normally, it must obtain sufficient yin fluids to moisten and
sprinkle it. Since the liver and kidneys have an especially close
relationship, kidney yin vacuity may easily result in liver yin vacuity
and loss of function of the liver qi. This is described as water failing
to moisten wood.

Water [may] not transform into qi. (水不化气 *Shui bu hua qi.*)
To understand the meaning of this statement, one must go back to
Tang Zong-hai's original explanation: Qi resides in [all] material
things, and [all material things eventually] revert to water. This is
clearly verifiable [from every day experience]. Indeed, the qi of the
human body is engendered below the navel within the cinnabar
field, [namely] the sea of qi. [The area] below the navel [is where]
the kidneys [and] the urinary bladder [are located], and this is
where water returns home to. This water does not itself transform
the qi but depends on the nose to inhale heavenly yang. Via the
lung passageways, heart fire is conducted downward to enter [the
space] below the navel, there to steam this water, [and it is this
which] promotes the transformation of qi. Just as [within] the (*I Jing
Classic of Change's*) trigram, *Kan* (water), one yang [line] is engendered from within water, so is the root of the engenderment of qi.

Water [may] not complement fire. (水不济火 *Shui bu ji huo.*)
The functions of water and fire within the body are mutually
dependent. Water controls fire and prevents fire from flaming
upward excessively, while fire transforms water with its warmth.
The word "complement" in this statement may also be translated as
to aid, help, relieve, or be of benefit to. Literally, *ji* means to cross
over a river. Kidney yin or water must travel upward to the heart to
keep heart fire under control.

[When] water is depleted, fire becomes effulgent. (水亏火旺
Shui kui huo wang.)
It is said that yin and yang in the body are nothing but fire and
water. As an extension of that, kidney yin vacuity may allow for
heart fire effulgence, while liver-kidney yin vacuity may allow for
liver fire effulgence or yang hyperactivity.

Miscellaneous five phase related sayings

The five qi enter the nose [and] are stored in the heart [and] lungs. (五气入鼻，藏于心肺。 *Wu qi ru bi, cang yu xin fei.*)
  The five qi are wind, cold, heat, dryness, and dampness.

The five flavors enter the mouth [and] are stored in the intestines [and] stomach. (五味入口，藏于肠胃。 *Wu wei ru kou, cang yu chang wei.*)
  The five flavors are the five flavors of food: sweet, sour, acrid, bitter, and salty.

LIFE PRINCIPLES, *i.e.*, PHYSIOLOGY
(生理 , *sheng li*)

In Chinese medicine, physiology means the functioning of the five viscera and six bowels, the qi, blood, fluids and humors, essence, and spirit, and the channels and network vessels.

The Five Viscera [and] Six Bowels
(五脏六腑, *wu zang liu fu*)

Liver, heart, spleen, lungs, [and] kidneys all pertain to yin [and] are the five viscera. Gallbladder, stomach, triple burner, urinary bladder, large intestine, [and] small intestine all pertain to yang [and] are the six bowels. (肝 心 脾 肺 肾皆属阴，五脏也。胆胃三焦膀胱大肠小肠皆属阳，六腑也。 *Gan xin pi fei shen jie shu yin, wu zang ye. Dan wei san jiao pang guang da chang xiao chang jie shu yang, liu fu ye.*)

The five viscera of Chinese medicine are the liver, heart, spleen, lungs, and kidneys. These all pertain to or are categorized as yin. The six bowels are the gallbladder, small intestine, stomach, large intestine, urinary bladder, and triple burner. These all are categorized as or pertain to yang.

The five viscera appear as one body. (五脏一体观。 *Wu zang yi ti guan.*)

While, in truth, the five viscera cannot be separated from the six bowels, the five viscera are sometimes seen as primary. What the above saying is implying is that the five viscera work together in order to produce one living human being.

The viscera [and] bowels are mutually connected. (脏腑相合 *Zang fu xiang he*)

This statement makes it clear that all the viscera and bowels are interconnected and mutually dependent. This is another statement of the thorough-going holism of Chinese medicine.

The viscera move qi to the bowels. (脏行气于腑 *Zang xing qi yu fu.*)

It is the viscera which engender the qi. Thus the bowels get their qi from their corresponding viscera. The bowels do not engender their own qi.

The bowels transport essence to the viscera. (腑输精于脏 *Fu shu jing yu zang.*)

The five viscera and six bowels all receive qi from the stomach. (五脏六腑皆禀气于胃 *Wu zang liu fu jie bing qi yu wei.*)

The stomach initiates the digestive process from which all latter heaven qi is produced in the body. While the stomach does not actually engender any qi, without the function of the stomach, there would be no place from which the other viscera and bowels could receive qi.

The six bowels fulfill their purpose when there is free flow. (六腑以通为用 *Liu fu yi tong wei yong.*)

The purpose of the bowels is to discharge turbidity or waste either from one bowel to the next, as in the stomach to small intestine to large intestine or from the body as in the large intestine and urinary bladder. This function of discharge can only occur if the qi of the bowels is freely flowing. Therefore, the bowels can only fulfill their purpose if their qi is freely flowing.

The five viscera transform humors. (五脏化液 *Wu zang hua ye.*)

Each of the five viscera transform one of the five humors. The liver transforms or makes tears, the heart transforms sweat, the spleen transforms drool, the lungs transform snivel (or nasal mucus), and the kidneys transform spittle.

The five viscera store [and] do not drain. (五脏藏而不泻 *Wu zang cang er bu xie.*)

The five viscera are replete. [They] store and do not drain. (五脏为实，藏而不泻 *Wu zang wei shi, cang er bu xie.*)

The five viscera store essence [and] qi and do not drain. Therefore, [they are] full but cannot be replete. (五脏者，藏精气而不泻也，故满而不能实。*Wu zang zhe, cang jing qi er bu xie ye, gu man er bu neng shi.*)

These four statements all make it clear that the five viscera store qi and essence and do not drain turbidity or waste like the bowels.

Humans have the five viscera to transform the five qi in order to engender joy, anger, sorrow, worry, [and] fear. (人有五脏化五气，以生喜怒悲忧恐。*Ren you wu zang hua wu qi, yi sheng xi nu bei you kong.*)

According to this statement, one of the functions of the five viscera is to experience consciousness or joy, anger, sorrow, worry, fear, etc. This is a clear statement of the concept of epiphenomenalism in Chinese medicine. Epiphenomenalism is the epistemological position that consciousness arises from the natural functioning of the human body.

The six bowels drain and do not store. (六腑泻不而藏 *Liu fu xie bu er cang.*)

The six bowels are empty. [They] drain and do not store. (六腑为空，泻而不藏 *Liu fu wei kong, xie er bu cang.*)

The six bowels convey [and] transform matter and do not store. (六腑传化物而不藏 *Liu fu chuan hua wu er bu cang.*)

The six bowels conduct and transform materials [and] do not store. Therefore, [they are] replete but are not able to be filled. (六腑者，传化物不藏，故实而不能满。*Liu fu zhe, chuan hua wu er bu cang, gu shi er bu neng man.*)

These four statements all make it clear that the six bowels drain and discharge turbidity or waste but they do not store qi or essence.

It is the free flow of the six bowels which make them function; [therefore,] flowing freely downward makes for [their] normalcy. (六腑以通为用，通下为顺。*Liu fu yi tong wei yong, tong xia wei shun.*)

[When] the six bowels are freely flowing, [they] are supplemented [*i.e.*, normally functioning]. (六腑以通为补。*Liu fu yi tong wei bu.*)

These two statements imply that the six bowels are normal and healthy as long as they flow freely. As a corollary of that, freeing the flow of the six bowels is a way to restore their health and well-being.

The eyes are the efflorescence of the five viscera [and] six bowels. (目是五脏六腑之精华。*Mu shi wu zang liu fu zhi jing hua.*)

The essence and qi of all the five viscera and six bowels are transmitted to the eyes. Therefore, the eyes may indicate the state of health of the five viscera and six bowels.

Liver
(肝, *gan*)

The liver pertains to wood. (肝属木 *Gan shu mu.*)

This means that the liver corresponds to the wood phase in five phase theory.

The liver is a yang viscus [which] is located in the middle burner. [It] is yang residing in yin. Therefore, it is yang within yin. (肝为阳脏，位于中焦，以阳居阴，故为阴中之阳也。*Gan wei yang zang, wei yu zhong jiao, yi yang ju yin, gu wei yin zhong zhi yang ye.*)

This statement describes the liver's anatomical location in terms of the three burners and also in terms of yin and yang relative to that location.

The liver's body is yin and its function is yang. (肝体阴而用阳 *Gan ti yin er yong yang.*)

> The liver's body or form is yin in that it is very soft and moist. However, the liver governs the coursing and discharge of the entire body. Therefore, its function is yang. Further, yang qi easily becomes replete and hyperactive within the liver.

The liver is the male viscus. (肝为牡脏 *Gan wei mu zang.*)

The liver is the unyielding [or indomitable] viscus. (肝为刚脏 *Gan wei gang zang.*)

> Both of these statements refer to the unyielding nature of the liver in terms of its function. It easily becomes depressed and its qi easily becomes stagnant. In that case, its qi is hard to move.

The liver is the unyielding viscus, the aiding of which consists of emolliating [it]. (肝为刚脏，济之以柔。 *Gan wei gang zang, ji zhi yi rou.*)

> This statement reiterates that the liver is the indomitable viscus. However, it goes on to say that the way to treat it is to emolliate it. This means to soften and relax the liver by nourishing liver blood.

The liver governs coursing [and] discharge. (肝主疏泄 *Gan zhu shu xie.*)

> The liver qi governs the coursing and discharge of the entire body. What this means is that the liver qi is what determines the lumen or openings of the various channels and vessels and bowels. If the liver qi is relaxed, then those lumena are relatively open and the associated vessel or bowel is freely flowing. However, if the liver qi is depressed, these lumena are constricted and the associated vessel or bowel is not freely flowing.

The liver [and] gallbladder together govern coursing [and] discharge. (肝胆同主疏泄。 *Gan dan tong zhu shu xie.*)

> This is a minor variation of the above statement. In this case, the author is stating that the liver and gallbladder work together to ensure coursing and discharge.

The liver stores the blood. (肝藏血 *Gan cang xue.*)
This means that, when the body is at rest or asleep, the blood
returns to the liver for storage. When the liver becomes active
again, the liver then releases the blood for use to the four
extremities.

The liver stores the blood [and] the heart moves it. A person's
stirring [or movement] leads to the blood moving through the
various channels. A person's stillness leads to the blood returning to the liver viscus. (肝藏血，心行之，人动则血运于诸
经，人静则血归于肝脏。 *Gan cang xue, xin xing zhi, ren dong
ze xue yun yu zhu jing, ren jing ze xue gui yu gan zang.*)

Because the liver pertains to wood [and] wood qi surges and
spreads, [if it] is not checked and depressed, the blood vessels
are freely and smoothly flowing. (以肝属木，木气冲和调达，
不致遏郁，则血脉痛畅。 *Yi gan shu mu, mu qi chong he tiao
da, bu zhi e yu, ze xue mai tong chang.*)
This statement implies the same thing as the saying, "The qi moves
the blood. If the qi moves, the blood moves. If the qi stops, the
blood stops." However, here, the movement of the qi is directly
and unambiguously related to the liver qi.

The liver is the viscus which stores the blood [and] also commands the ministerial fire. (肝为藏血之脏，又司相火。 *Gan
wei zang xue zhi zang, you si xiang huo.*)
Above we have seen that the liver stores the blood. However, the
liver also has a specially close relationship to the life-gate/ministerial
fire. If ministerial fire flames (炎, *yan*) or stirs (动, *dong*) upward, this
may cause or aggravate depressive heat. *Vice versa*, depresssive
heat in the liver may cause ministerial fire to stir upward.

The liver governs the sinews. (肝主筋 *Gan zhu jin.*)
The sinews are the tissue that corresponds to the liver according to
five phase theory. Therefore, it is said that the liver governs the
sinews. In particular, it is liver blood which nourishes the sinews,
allowing them to move freely and extend freely.

When the liver obtains blood, the sinews are soothed. (肝的得血
则筋舒 *Gan de de xue ze jin shu.*)

Because the sinews are nourished by liver blood, when the liver
obtains sufficient blood, the sinews are able to stretch and extend
normally. *Vice versa,* if the liver blood is vacuous and the sinews do
not obtain their proper nourishment, the sinews become dry and
tend to contract or spasm.

The liver governs fright. (肝主惊 *Gan zhu jing.*)

This saying is not so easy to explain briefly. In ancient China, there
were two competing ideas about courage. On the one hand, courage was an expression of abundant heart qi. On the other, courage
was the expression of a freely flowing and healthy gallbladder and
the gallbladder receives its qi from the liver. Even today, we say that
a person who is very forward "has a lot of gall." This is based on
this same ancient idea that bile or gall is somehow associated with
having courage or being brave.

Anger is the orientation [*i.e.,* emotion or affect] of the liver.
(肝志为怒 *Gan zhi wei nu.*)

The liver governs anger. (肝主怒 *Gan zhu nu.*)

Anger damages the liver. (怒伤肝 *Nu shang gan.*)

All three of these statements relate anger to the liver. The cor-
relation between anger and the liver is based on five phase theory
correspondences and the five orientations or affects. However, this
relationship between anger and the liver is bidirectional. Anger is
the subjective experience of liver depression, but, *vice versa,* great
anger or explosive anger damages the liver.

Qi depression damages the liver. (气郁伤肝。 *Qi yu shang gan.*)

Qi depression is the fundamental internally engendered disease
mechanism of the liver. When qi depression damages the liver, it
may evolve into depressive liver heat, ascendant liver yang
hyperactivity, liver fire flaming upward, and the last two of these
may evolve into internal stirring of liver wind.

The liver qi easily [becomes] depressed [and] easily
counterflows. (肝气易郁，易逆。 *Gan qi yi yu, yi ni.*)

This is yet another statement about how liver depression qi stagnation easily occurs and then easily leads to complications.

The liver governs the sea of blood. (肝主血海 *Gan zhu xue hai.*)

The sea of blood is the *chong mai* (冲脉) or penetrating vessel. Since the liver governs the storage of blood, it is also said that the liver governs the sea of blood. In clinical practice, this saying is commonly used to help explain meno- and metrorrhagia as the liver's failure to properly govern the sea of blood.

The liver is the sea of blood. (肝为血海 *Gan wei xue hai.*)

This statement goes even further than the preceding statement, simply equating the liver with the sea of blood. This helps explain the close relationship between the liver and the *chong mai.*

The blood chamber is the liver. (血室者肝也。 *Xue shi zhe gan ye.*)

The blood chamber is another name for the uterus. This statement further underscores the importance of the liver to menstruation and fertility.

The liver governs [physical] movement. (肝主运动 *Gan zhu yun dong.*)

Movement is nothing other than the expression of the movement of qi, and this movement of qi is dependent on the liver's governing over coursing and discharge. If the liver qi is smoothly (畅, *chang*) and freely (通, *tong*) flowing, then coursing and discharge are normal and the body's qi is also freely and smoothly flowing.

The liver governs upbearing [and] effusion. (肝主升发 *Gan zhu sheng fa.*)

The coursing and discharge of the liver qi governs the uninhibited (不利, *bu li*) and free flow of the qi mechanism or dynamic (气机, *qi ji*). The qi mechanism controls the four movements of the qi: upbearing (升, *sheng*), exiting (出, *chu*), downbearing (降, *jiang*), and entering (入, *ru*). However, because liver yang commonly has a surplus and yang qi tends to move upward in the body, the liver especially governs upbearing and exiting or effusing.

The liver governs the interior of the entire body. (肝主一身之里 *Gan zhu yi shen zhi li.*)

> This saying is a parallel saying to the lungs' governing the exterior of the entire body. Together, the liver and lungs govern the movement of the qi of the entire body. The lungs provide the motivating power, while the liver controls the lumena of the channels and vessels through which the qi moves. In particular, the lungs govern the movement of the defensive qi (卫气, *wei qi*) through the exterior of the body. By extension then, the implication of this saying is that the liver governs the constructive qi (营气, *ying qi*) which primarily moves on the interior of the body.

The liver is averse to wind. (肝恶风 *Gan wu feng.*)

> According to five phase theory, wood corresponds to wind and the liver corresponds to wood. In clinical practice, this statement means that wind can aggravate liver conditions. For instance, migraine headaches are typically ascribed to the liver, and migraines are often initiated or aggravated by windy weather.

The liver is the wind viscus. (肝为风脏 *Gan wei feng zang.*)

> This means three things. First, the liver is the wood viscus and wood corresponds to wind. Secondly, it means that the liver is easily damaged by wind as explained above. Third, it also means that liver disease may give rise to the internal engenderment of wind stirring in the body, as in stroke and other forms of paralysis and spasticity.

The liver is the viscus of wind [and] wood. (肝为风木之脏 *Gan wei feng mu zhi zang.*)

The liver governs wind. (肝主风 *Gan zhu feng.*)

> These two sayings only further reiterate the foregoing. In particular, the last statement means that internally stirring wind is engendered by or within the liver.

The corresponding warm qi of spring nourishes the liver. (应春温之气以养肝. *Ying chun wen zhi qi yi yang gan.*)

> The warm qi of spring is relaxing to the liver after the constricting cold of winter.

The liver holds the office of general and strategies emanate from there. (肝者, 将军之官, 谋虑出焉 *Gan zhe, jiang jun zhi guan, mou lu chu yan.*)

> According to the theory within the *Nei Jing (Inner Classic)* likening each of the five viscera and six bowels to officials within the imperial bureaucracy, the liver is like a general who is in charge of long-term or strategic planning. Therefore, inability to plan long-term is sometimes ascribed to the liver. However, this statement is not so commonly met nowadays.

The liver governs the making of strategies. (肝主谋虑 *Gan zhu mou lu.*)

> This statement reiterates that the ability to strategize is associated with the function of the liver.

The liver stores the ethereal soul. (肝藏魂 *Gan cang hun.*)

> In ancient China as in many ancient cultures, the psyche was made up of a number of different semi-independent entities. Therefore, there was the spirit (神, *shen*), the ethereal soul (魂, *hun*), and the corporeal soul (魄, *po*). The ethereal soul in particular was that part of the psyche that wandered during sleep in the dreamland. According to five phase theory, this ethereal soul is stored in the liver.

The liver has its efflorescence in the nails. (肝气华在爪 *Gan qi hua zai zhao.*)

The nails are the surplus of the sinews. (爪为筋之余 *Zhao wei jin zhi yu.*)

> Both of these two statements have to do with the five phase correspondences between wood, the liver, the sinews, and the nails. Liver blood nourishes the sinews. If this causes a surplus of the sinews, then this surplus grows into the nails. Therefore, the health and vigor of the nails reflect the state of liver blood.

The liver lives on the left. (肝生于左 *Gan zhu yu zuo.*)

> This statement is clearly anatomically wrong. However, it has to do with the dualism between the liver and the lungs. Both these two viscera control the qi within the body. Since it is said that the lungs live on the right, the liver must then live on the left.

The liver engenders [or arises] on the left, [while] the lungs store on the right. (肝生于左，肺藏于右。 *Gan sheng yu zuo, fei cang yu you.*)
> This statement asserts a reciprocal relationship between the liver and lungs associated with the right and left sides respectively.

Upbearing on the left side of people's bodies pertains to the liver. (人身左升属肝 *Ren shen zuo sheng shu gan.*)
> This statement is perhaps more understandable than the previous one. Rather than saying that the liver is anatomically located on the left, it says that the upbearing on the left pertains to the liver. This statement is often used to explain left-sided hadaches due to upward counterflow of the liver qi.

Blood nourishes the hair. (血养发 *Xue yang fa.*)

Hair is the surplus of the blood. (发为血之余 *Fa wei xue zhi yu.*)
> Just as the blood nourishes the sinews and the nails are the surplus of the sinews, the hair is the surplus of the blood. Therefore, the state of the hair is also an indication of the state of liver blood. In particular, graying and/or loss of the head hair are both associated with a liver blood vacuity.

The liver [and] kidneys [are of or share] a common source. (肝肾同源 *Gan shen tong yuan.*)
> The liver and kidneys share an especially close relationship. As we have seen above, the liver is closely associated with life gate/ ministerial fire which is rooted in kidney yang or fire. In addition, liver blood and kidney essence are closely associated. A surplus of blood is necessary in order to make latter heaven essence, while some kidney essence is also necessary in order to engender and transform blood. Therefore, it is said that the liver and kidneys share a common source.

The liver [and] kidneys are mutually engendering. (肝肾相生 *Gan shen xiang sheng.*)
> Kidney yin nourishes and moistens the liver, while kidney yang warms and steams the liver. However, liver blood helps make kidney essence, and essence can be transformed into either yin or yang.

The liver [and] kidneys, these two, both command the lower burner. (肝与肾二者同司下焦。 *Gan yu shen er zhe tong si xia jiao.*)
> This means that lower burner diseases are mostly associated with the liver and/or kidneys.

The liver pulse is bowstring. (肝脉弦 *Gan mai xian.*)[1]
> According to five phase theory, the liver pulse is bowstring or wiry. This wiry feeling reflects the constriction in the channels and vessels due to the liver's failure to govern coursing and discharge properly.

[If one] presses [and feels] bowstring, [this] is the liver vessel. All pain pertains to the liver, and the jue yin vessel traverses the lesser abdomen. (按弦为肝脉，诸痛属肝, 厥阴之脉循少腹。 *An xian wei gan mai, zhu tong shu gan, jue yin zhi mai xun shao fu.*)
> This statement confirms that the liver pulse is the bowstring or wiry pulse. However, it also implies that a bowstring pulse may indicate a lower abdominal disease since the jue yin liver channel traverses the liver.

The liver qi flows to the eyes. (肝气通于目 *Gan qi tong yu mu.*)
> This statement explains the liver's anatomical relationship to the eyes via an internal channel.

The liver opens into the orifices of the eyes. (肝开窍于目 *Gan kai qiao yu mu.*)
> According to five phase theory, the liver and eyes correspond. Therefore, in Chinese medicine, vision problems tend to be ascribed to disorders of the liver.

[When] the liver receives blood, there is the ability to see. (肝受血而能视 *Gan shou xue er neng shi.*)

---

[1] According to Wiseman *et al.*, 弦 (*xian*) should be translated as "string-like." However, a string may be either taught or loose, but here, this word specifically implies the tension of a strung bowstring. Many English-speakers use the word "wiry." However, the Chinese character shows a bow, and bows use strings not wires.

According to the *Nei Jing (Inner Classic)*, the qi of any and all tissues and organs in the body can only perform its function as long as that tissue or organ is nourished by adequate blood. The function (用, *yong*) of the eyes are to see, and the eyes correspond and are connected to the liver. Therefore, the eyes can only see when the liver obtains sufficient blood to nourish them.

[When] the liver is harmonious, the eyes are able to differentiate the five colors. (肝和则眼能辨五色 *Gan he ze yan neng bian wu se.*)

This statement likewise relates proper visual function of the eyes to the healthy and normal function of the liver.

The liver forms the tears. (肝为泪 *Gan wei lei.*)

Tears are the liver humor. (泪为肝液 *Lei wei gan ye.*)

Both these two statements have to do with the five phase correspondence between the liver and tears, the tears being the humor of the liver. However, this does not mean necessarily that crying has mostly to do with the liver. It is specifically tears which correspond to the liver, not the act of crying.

Food qi enters the stomach; it disperses essence to the liver [and] licentious qi to the sinews. (食气入胃，散精于肝，淫气于筋 *Shi qi ru wei, san jing yu gan, yin qi yu jin.*)

While this statement starts with the stomach, it mainly concerns the liver and the liver's relationship to sexual performance in the male. The penis is referred to as the gathering or reunion of the sinews. That this statement is talking about the penis and its ability to engage in intercourse is indicated by the word "licentious." What this statement means is that the finest essence of food and drink transformed by the spleen is necessary for the liver to nourish the sinews adequately, including the penis, in order for the penis to be able to engage in intercourse.

The knees are the mansion of the sinews.[2] (膝为筋之府 *Xi wei jin zhi fu.*)

---

[2] Wiseman *et al.* translate 府 (*fu*) simply as "house." However, the Chinese word refers not just to anyone's house but to an official residence. In

Normally, in Chinese medicine, the knees are thought of corresponding to the kidneys. However, this statement says that the
knees are the mansion of the sinews. Since the sinews correspond
to the liver, the state of the knees must also be closely related to
the liver. In fact, in clinical practice, we often have to treat the liver
for knee problems, not just the kidneys.

All the sinews home to the joints. (诸筋者，皆属于节。 *Zhu jin zhe, jie shu yu jie.*)

This statement makes it clear that the sinews attach to the joints
and play a part in the movement of the joints. If the sinews are
nourished and moistened properly, they can extend. However, if
they become dry and malnourished, they contract and cannot
extend properly. It is specifically liver blood that nourishes and
moistens the sinews.

[At] seven [times] eight [years, *i.e.,* 56], the liver qi is debilitated [and] the sinews are not able to stir. (七八肝气衰，筋不能动。 *Qi ba gan qi shuai, jin bu neng dong.*)

This statement makes explicit what the previous statement only
implies, that the liver and kidneys are both typically involved in
disorders of the knees.

[In] women, the liver is the former heaven. (女子以肝为先天 *Nu zi yi gan wei xian tian.*)

Normally, in Chinese medicine, we say that the kidneys are the
former heaven viscus because the kidneys store former heaven
essence. But above we have seen that the liver stores the blood
and blood and essence share a common source. Because the
menstruate is the outward manifestation of the essence in women
and the liver helps control the amount of the menstruate via the
chong mai, the liver is just as important as the kidneys when it
comes to understanding the menstrual cycle and female fertility.
Therefore, it is not that the liver is the former heaven in women
and the kidneys are not but that the liver and kidneys must be
taken together as the former heaven in females.

American English, we speak about the governor's mansion and the mayor's
mansion. Therefore, I prefer to translate this word as "mansion."

The blacks of the eyes are the essence of the liver. (肝之精为黑眼　*Gan zhi jing wei hei yan.*)
This means that the state of the blacks of the eyes may indicate the state of liver yin, blood, and essence.

The liver vessel networks with the root of the tongue. (肝脉络于舌本　*Gan mai luo yu she ben.*)
This statement says that a network vessel from the liver connects with the root of the tongue and, therefore, the liver must be taken into account in tongue and speech problems, for instance in deviation of the tongue due to wind stroke.

The liver vessel networks with the yin organs. (肝脉络阴器 *Gan mai luo yin qi.*)
Yin here refers to the genitals. Thus, the liver channel surrounds the genitals. Therefore, all problems with the genitals may be due to problems with the liver.

The liver is delighted by orderly reaching. (肝喜条达　*Gan xi tiao da.*)
This means that the liver qi is normal when it is freely flowing and able to promote the coursing and discharge of the entire body. Conversely, when the liver qi is not able to spread freely, it becomes depressed and diseased.

The green-blue color pertains to the liver. (青色属肝　*Qing se shu gan.*)
This is a five phase correspondence between the wood phase, the liver viscus, and the green-blue color. In clinical practice, a green-blue color of the face often indicates a liver disorder.

The sour flavor enters the liver. (酸味入肝　*Suan wei ru gan.*)
This is another five phase correspondence between wood, the liver, and the sour flavor. Often, medicinals which are meant to enter the liver are stir-fried in vinegar so that the sour flavor of the vinegar acts as a guide leading the medicinal more efficiently into that viscus. A sour taste in the mouth may also indicate a liver disorder.

The liver rules the spring. (肝主春　*Gan zhu chun.*)
According to five phase theory, wood, the liver, and the spring time all correspond. Interestingly, a number of diseases which Chinese

medicine relates to the liver are aggravated or recur in the spring, such as cluster headaches.

The corresponding warm qi of spring nourishes the liver. (应春温之气以养肝. *Ying chun wen zhi qi yi yang gan.*)

Because the liver corresponds to the spring via the wood phase, the liver is typically strong during this time. If it is a healthy strength, then there is good health. However, the liver tends to have a surplus. Therefore, often, spring leads to various yang repletions.

The liver is the source of the constructive. (肝为营之源 *Gan wei yin zhi yuan.*)

Because the liver stores the blood and the blood is the mother of the qi, the liver is the source of the constructive qi. If liver blood is insufficient, the constructive qi cannot be healthy and exuberant.

The liver vessel traverses both sides of the body. (肝脉行身之两旁 *Gan mai xing shen zhi liang pang.*)

The liver and gallbladder channels both traverse the rib-side of the body. Therefore, one-sided or specifically costal complaints are often associated with liver-gallbladder disorders.

The rib-sides are the boundaries of the liver. (胁为肝之分也 *Xie wei gan zhi fen ye.*)

This statement basically means the foregoing, that problems in the rib-sides and hypochondrium are commonly related to the liver.

[If] the liver is obstructed, both rib-sides [are] painful. (肝壅，两胁痛。 *Gan yong, liang xie tong.*)

This is a corollary of the above two statements.

The sinews are the liver's conjunction. (筋者肝之合 *Jin zhe gan zhi he.*)

This saying means that the places where the sinews join or attach have an especially close relationship to liver blood. If the liver fails to nourish the sinews in these areas adequately, soreness and pain may occur with eventual loss of function.

The liver is united with the gallbladder. (肝合胆 *Gan he dan.*)

The liver [and] gallbladder [stand in] a mutual exterior/interior [relationship]. (肝与胆相表里 *Gan yu dan xiang biao li.*)
> These two sayings indicate that the liver and gallbladder have a yin-yang, interior-exterior relationship. The gallbladder gets its qi from the liver, and problems in the liver can reflect or manifest along the gallbladder channel.

[If] the liver offends, its nature [consists of] lots of stirring and little stillness, [and it] easily assails some other viscus. (肝者干也，其性多动而少静，好干犯他脏。 *Gan zhe gan ye, qi xing duo dong er shao jing, hao gan fan ta zang.*)
> This statement means two things. First, if liver yang becomes hyperactive, it causes lots of stirring and little stillness as in internal stirring of liver wind. Secondly, when the liver becomes diseased, it easily causes disease in any other of the five viscera and six bowels. For instance, liver-stomach, liver-spleen, liver-lung, liver-heart, liver-kidney, and liver-large intestine disharmonies are all commonly seen in clinical practice.

All wind [with] shaking and dizziness pertains to the liver. (诸风掉眩，皆属于肝。 *Zhu feng diao xuan, jie shu yu gan.*)
> This statement is a more succinct reiteration of the first half of the previous statement.

The liver is the root of congealed [*i.e.*, static] blood. (肝者，凝血之本。 *Gan zhe, ning xue zhi ben.*)
> This is because the qi moves the blood. Therefore, liver depression qi stagnation easily results in the creation of blood stasis over time.

Ministerial fire attaches [itself] internally [within] the liver. (肝内寄相火。 *Gan nei ji xiang huo.*)

Fire attaches within the liver-gallbladder. (肝胆火寄于中。 *Gan dan huo ji yu zhong.*)
> These two statements emphasize the close relationship between the liver and life-gate/ministerial fire.

The liver is the thief of the five viscera [and] six bowels. (肝为五脏六腑之贼。 *Gan wei wu zang liu fu zhi zei.*)

This statement means that the liver is the most commonly diseased of all the five viscera and six bowels. This is because liver depression qi stagnation is so common. In this saying, the word 贼 (*zei*) means thief, traitor, enemy, or the wicked or evil one.

Gallbladder
(胆, *dan*)

The gallbladder governs decisions. (胆主决断 *Dan zhu jue duan.*)

This means that the gallbladder governs short-term decisions as opposed to the liver's governing long-term strategies. Therefore, inability to make decisions is sometimes seen as indicating a gallbladder disease.

The gallbladder is the mansion of clear fluid; inside it is lodged ministerial fire. (胆为清津之府，内寄相火 *Gan wei qing jin zhi fu, nei ji xiang huo.*)

The clear fluid referred to here is bile. The second part of this statement refers to the particularly close relationship of the liver and gallbladder to ministerial fire.

The gallbladder is *shao yang* ministerial fire. (胆为少阳相火。 *Dan wei shao yang xiang huo.*)

The gallbladder [has] within [it] ministerial fire. (胆中相火。 *Dan zhong xiang huo.*)

The gallbladder commands ministerial fire. (胆司相火。 *Dan si xiang huo.*)

These three statements likewise assert an especially close relationship between the gallbladder and ministerial fire.

The gallbladder [is] the mansion of the central essence. (胆者，中精之府。 *Dan zhe, zhong jing zhi fu.*)

The central essence spoken of in this statement is the bile which the gallbladder stores and discharges.

The gallbladder vessel networks with the ear. (胆脉络于耳 *Dan mai luo yu er.*)
The course of the foot *shao yang* gallbladder channel surrounds the outer ear. Therefore, disorders of the liver-gallbladder may result in ear and hearing disorders.

The gallbladder [and] the liver [have] the same palace. (肝胆同宫 *Gan dan tong gong.*)
The gallbladder is located snug up against the liver. Therefore, it may be said that they share or have the same palace or abode.

The 11 viscera depend on the gallbladder. (十一脏取决于胆 *Shi yi zang qu jue yu dan.*)
The 11 viscera refer to the remaining five viscera and five bowels. The secretion of bile is an important part of the digestive process from which the qi and blood of all the other viscera and bowels comes.

[If] the qi makes for a strong gallbladder, evils cannot attack. (气以胆壮，邪不可干。 *Qi yi dan zhuang, xie bu ke gan.*)
This statement has to do with the gallbladder's role in the engenderment and transformation of qi and blood.

Heart
(心, *xin*)

The heart pertains to fire. (心属火 *Xin shu huo.*)
This means that the heart corresponds to the fire phase within five phase theory.

The heart is sovereign fire [which] transforms [and] engenders blood. (心为君火，化生血液。 *Xin wei jun huo, hua sheng xue ye.*)
In Chinese medicine, there are two types of fire within the body. The first is sovereign fire (君火, *jun huo*) or heart fire. The second is ministerial fire (相火, *xiang huo*). Ministerial fire is the fire of the life-gate which is rooted in the lower burner. These two fires are mutually connected, but, within the body, sovereign fire is supreme. Within five phase theory, sovereign fire also encompasses the small

intestines, while ministerial fire is also the pericardium or heart ruler and the triple burner. We will deal with the heart's relationship to the blood below.

Heart fire is sovereign fire; liver [and] kidney fire is ministerial fire. (心火为君火，肝肾之火为相火。 *Xin huo wei jun huo, gan shen zhi huo wei xiang huo.*)

This is a slightly different statement about sovereign and ministerial fires. Ministerial fire can also be said to be rooted in kidney yang or kidney fire, and, although ministerial fire does ligate or communicate with all the tissues and organs of the body, the liver has an especially close relationship to life-gate/ministerial fire.

The heart wrapper network vessels [*i.e.*, the pericardium] are ministerial fire. (心包络为相火。 *Xin bao luo wei xiang huo.*)

This statement identifies the pericardium with the ministerial fire.

The heart governs the blood. (心主血 *Xin zhu xue.*)

The heart's governing of the blood means that it is the heart qi which stirs or propels the blood through the vessels. In addition, the heart plays a part in the engenderment of the blood, turning it red before it is sent out into the vessels.

The heart's talent is also to govern the engenderment of blood. (心之能事，又主生血。 *Xin zhi neng shi, you zhu sheng xue.*)

As stated above, the heart plays the final role in the engenderment and transformation of the blood. The spleen sends the finest essence of food and drink upward. While the kidneys send essence upward as well, it is the heart qi which combines the finest essence of food and drink with this kidney essence and turns it red, thus becoming the finished product of blood.

All blood homes to the heart. (诸血者，皆属于心。 *Zhu xue zhe, jie shu yu xin.*)

This is a recognition that all the blood vessels home to or connect with the heart and that all the blood flows through the heart in its circulation throughout the body.

The heart is the root of the constructive [and] defensive. (心者，营卫之本。 *Xin zhe, ying wei zhi ben.*)

The constructive and the defensive are both species of qi. However, the heart governs the blood and the blood is the mother of the qi. Therefore, from this point of view, one can say that the heart is the root of the constructive and the defensive.

The heart governs the spirit light. (心主神明 *Xin zhu shen ming.*)

The heart stores the spirit. (心藏神 *Xin cang shen.*)

These two statements imply that the heart is the seat of consciousness in the human body. Within contemporary Chinese medicine, there are two theories about consciousness. One theory is called the heart-ruling theory and the other theory is called the brain-ruling theory. According to this second theory, introduced by Li Shi-zhen in the Ming dynasty, the brain is the organ of or seat of consciousness within the body. The above two statements are examples of the heart-ruling theory, the original theory of consciousness within Chinese medicine.

The heart holds the office of monarch from whence the spirit light emanates. (心者君主之官也，神明出焉 *Xin zhe jun zhu zhi guan ye, shen ming chu yan.*)

This statement similarly implies that the heart is the seat of consciousness. However, it also says that, within the body, the heart is the supreme monarch.

The heart is the great ruler of the five viscera [and] six bowels, the place of abode of the essence spirit. (心者，五脏六腑之大主也，精神之所舍也。 *Xin zhe, wu zang liu fu zhi da zhu ye, jing shen zhi suo she ye.*)

This statement reiterates the two points of the previous statement: 1) that the heart is the sovereign within the body and 2) that the heart governs the psyche. In Chinese, essence spirit (精神, *jing shen*) as a compound term means psyche or the mental-emotional functions.

The place from which things are appointed is called the heart. (所以任物者谓之心。 *Suo yi ren wu zhe wei zhi xin.*)

This is yet again a statement that the heart is the sovereign within the body since ultimately it was the emperor within the Chinese political hierarchy who was responsible for governmental appointments.

[It is] not ok for the heart [to be] damaged. (心不可伤。 *Xin bu ke shang.*)

> Because the heart is supreme within the body, it is not ok for the heart to be damaged. Damage of the heart viscus may lead to the heart stopping beating, and cessation of the heart's beating signals death.

Thought exits from the heart and the spleen responds [to it]. (思出于心，而脾应之。 *Si chu yu xin, er pi ying zhi.*)

> This statement makes it clear that, at least according to the heart-ruling theory of consciousness, thought is a function of the heart to which the spleen only responds.

The heart governs the vessels. (心主脉 *Xin zhu mai.*)

The heart governs the blood [and] vessels. (心主血脉 *Xin zhu xue mai.*)

> In Chinese medicine, the word "vessels" (脉, *mai*), as opposed to "channels" (经, *jing*) typically means the blood vessels and the blood vessels are governed by the heart.

The heart governs speech. (心主言 *Xin zhu yan.*)

> This statement relates the coherence and quality of the speech to the heart. For instance, deranged speech or delirium indicates a disquieted heart spirit, while normal coherent or logical speech indicates a normal, healthy heart spirit.

The heart opens into the orifice of the tongue. (心开窍于舌 *Xin kai qiao yu she.*)

The tongue is the sprout of the heart. (舌为心之苗 *She wei xin zhi miao.*)

> These two statements indicate that the tongue as a whole corresponds to the heart. This includes both the speech produced by the tongue and physical changes in the appearance of the tongue, both of which may indicate disorders of the heart.

If the heart is harmonious, the tongue is able to know [*i.e.*, distinguish] flavors. (心和则舌能知味 *Xin he ze she neng zhi wei.*)

This statement is based on five phase theory. The tongue is the organ of taste which corresponds to the heart. Therefore, inability to taste reflects a heart disorder. However, this statement is not commonly invoked today. Instead, inability to taste is more commonly ascribed to spleen vacuity.

The vessel of the heart fastens to the root of the tongue. (心之脉系于舌本 *Xin zhi mai xi yu she ben.*)

This statement explains how the heart connects to the tongue via the channels and network vessels.

The heart has its efflorescence in the face. (心气华在面 *Xin qi hua zai mian.*)

This means that the facial complexion may reflect the condition of the heart, and certainly a normal rosy complexion indicates a healthy circulatory system. In particular, a face which is too red indicates heat, including heat in the heart, while a pale face indicates blood vacuity, including heart blood vacuity.

The heart is averse to heat. (心恶热 *Xin wu re.*)

All heat in the body tends to float upward to the heart and lungs, and heat evils may cause the heart qi or spirit to stir or move frenetically, thus causing psychological disorders. Therefore, even though the heart corresponds to fire according to five phase theory, the heart is averse to heat.

The corresponding hot qi of summer nourishes the heart. (应夏热之气以养心。 *Ying xia re zhi qi yi yang xin.*)

This statement would seem to contradict the previous one. However, the implication of the present statement is that the normal warmth of summer promotes the free and easy flow of the heart qi and blood and, therefore, is good for the heart. It is only excessive heat that damages the heart.

The qi of summer communicates with the heart. (夏气通于心 *Xia qi tong yu xin.*)

This statement indicates that both the summer and the heart correspond to the fire phase in five phase theory. Therefore, the qi of summer (*i.e.*, its weather) affects the heart. As long as this qi is not too hot, the warmth of summer benefits heart function as stated above.

Turbid qi goes to the heart. (浊气归心 *Zhuo qi gui xin.*)
This statement is usually interpreted to mean that the turbid part of
the clear goes to or gathers in the heart where it becomes the
blood. To understand this concept, we must know that, just like yin
and yang, clear and turbid each can be subdivided into clear and
turbid. Thus the clear of the clear goes to the lungs to become the
qi, while the turbid of the clear goes to the heart to become the
blood.

Joy is the orientation [*i.e.*, emotion or affect] of the heart. (心志
为喜 *Xin zhi wei xi.*)
In Chinese medicine, joy can mean either of two things. First, it can
mean a state of hyperexcitation. In this case, an excess of joy causes
frenetic movement of the heart qi with disquietude of the spirit.
Secondly, joy can mean happiness (乐, *le*). Happiness makes for
relaxtion. Thus happiness can be the antidote to all the other affects.
However, when happiness is excessive, too much relaxation may
lead to slowing of movement of the heart qi and, therefore, blood.

The heart desires softness [*i.e.*, stillness, calmness, or quiet].
(心欲软。*Xin yu ruan.*)
"Softness" in this statement implies stillness (静, *jing*), calmness (宁,
ning), and quiet (安, *an*). The heart spirit is healthy when it is calm
and quiet. In other words, although the heart qi or spirit must move,
it should not move too much. Rather, it should move softly or
calmly.

Sweat is the heart humor. (汗为心液 *Han wei xin ye.*)
Among the five humors, sweat is the humor that corresponds to
the heart. In terms of clinical practice, spontaneous sweating may
indicate a heart qi vacuity, while night sweats may indicate a heart
yin and blood vacuity.

The heart pulse is surging. (心脉洪 *Xin mai hong.*)
The surging pulse is a large (*i.e.*, wide), forceful, floating pulse,
especially in the inch position. While a moderately surging pulse is
normal in the inch position, an excessively surging pulse indicates
heart fire effulgence due to yin failing to control yang. Instead, yang
floats upwards and outwards, creating the floating and large pulse.

The color red pertains to the heart. (赤色属心 *Chi se shu xin.*)

Red is the color corresponding to the fire phase as well as the color of blood. Therefore, a red facial complexion or red skin lesions may indicate heat evils accumulated in the heart. Similarly, fresh red blood may indicate heat in the blood aspect which may also damage the heart since the heart governs the blood.

The bitter flavor enters the heart. (苦味入心 *Ku wei ru xin.*)

According to five phase theory, the bitter flavor corresponds to the fire phase as does the heart. Therefore, it is believed that the bitter flavor enters the heart from which it drains and discharges heat evils.

The upper back is yang, [and] the heart is yang within yang. (背为阳，阳中之阳心也。 *Bei wei yang, yang zhong zhi yang xin ye.*)

This statement explains the heart's physical location in terms of yin-yang theory.

The heart [and] spleen [are] mutually involved. (心脾相关。 *Xin pi xiang guan.*)

The spleen is the source of both the heart qi and blood. The finest essence of food and drink is sent upward by the spleen to become the heart qi (the clear of the clear) via the lungs and the blood (the turbid of the clear). *Vice versa*, emotional upsets affecting the heart may also affect spleen function.

The heart [and] kidneys mutually interact. (心肾相交 *Xin shen xiang jiao.*)

The heart [and] kidneys mutually interact, [and] their upbearing [and] downbearing depend on each other. The heart qi's downbearing causes the kidney qi's upbearing, [while] the kidney qi's upbearing also causes the heart qi's downbearing. (心肾相交，全凭升降。而心气之降，由于肾气之升；肾气之升，又因心气之降。 *Xin shen xiang jiao, quan ping sheng jiang. Er xin qi zhi jiang, you yu shen qi zhi sheng; shen qi zhi sheng, you yin xin qi zhi jiang.*)

The interaction between the heart and kidneys is the interaction between fire and water in the body. The heart qi must descend to transform kidney water. However, kidney water must ascend to control heart fire and keep it from flaming or flaring upward hyperactively.

The heart is united with the small intestine. (心合小肠 *Xin he xiao chang.*)

According to five phase theory, the heart and small intestine both correspond to the fire phase. In that case, the heart is the yin fire viscus and the small intestine is the yang fire bowel. In clinical practice, heat evils in the heart can be transmitted to the small intestine. This is because heat is yang and has no inherent affinity for such a yin viscus. Therefore, the yang heat flows naturally to the yang bowel where there is a yin-yang affinity.

The heart [and] small intestine [stand in or have] a mutual interior-exterior [relationship]. (心与小肠相表里 *Xin yu xiao chang xiang biao li.*)

Based on a combination of both five phase and yin-yang theory, the relationship of the heart to the small intestine is called an interior-exterior relationship. In this case, the heart is interior and the small intestine is exterior.

The chest center [or *dan zhong*] is the palace wall of the heart ruler. (膻中者，心主之宫城。 *Dan zhong zhe, xin zhu zhi gong cheng.*)

This statement makes it clear that the *dan zhong* is another name for the pericardium or heart ruler.

The chest is the official of feudal messengers [from which] exit joy [and] happiness. (膻者，使臣之官，喜乐出也。 *Dan zhe, shi chen zhi guan, xi le chu ye.*)

Here the word for the chest is 膻 (*dan*) as in *dan zhong*, chest center. In this statement, it refers to the heart and lungs together, and the statement suggests that happiness and joy exit from this part of the body.

Small Intestine
(小肠, *xiao chang*)

The small intestine governs the separation of the clear from the turbid. (小肠主分清别浊 *Xin chang zhu fen qing bie zhuo.*)

The small intestine receives the remainder of the digestate from the stomach.

The small intestine transforms food [and] separates the clear from the turbid. (小肠化食，分别清浊 *Xiao chang hua shi, fen bie qing zhuo.*)

Remember that clear and turbid can also each be further separated into clear and turbid. Therefore, when this statement says that the small intestine separates the clear from the turbid, it means that it separates the clear of the turbid from the turbid of the turbid. The clear from the turbid is reabsorbed, while the turbid of the turbid is sent down to the large intestine for excretion.

The small intestine governs humors. (小肠主液 *Xiao chang zhu ye.*)

According to this statement, the small intestine reabsorbs those fluids from food and drink that become the humors in the body. The humors in the body are the thick fluids, such as the intra-articular fluids and cerebrospinal fluids.

The small intestine is the official of receiving plenitude; materials are transformed [and] exit here. (小肠者受盛之官，化物出焉 *Xiao chang zhe shou sheng zhi guan, hua wu chu yan.*)

This statement basically reiterates the foregoing statements in terms of the small intestine's roles. However, in contemporary Chinese medicine, little clinically is made of the small intestine. In fact, small intestine vacuity has been collapsed into spleen qi vacuity, the only difference being the presence of marked borborygmus in small intestine vacuity.

The small intestine governs urination. (小肠主小便。*Xiao chang zhu xiao bian.*)

The turbid fluids separated by the small intestine are sent down to the kidneys and bladder for transformation into urine and discharged from the body. That is why this statement says the small intestine governs urination.

Spleen
(脾, *pi*)

The spleen pertains to earth. (脾属土 *Pi shu tu.*)
This means that, according to five phase theory, the spleen corresponds to the earth phase.

[If] spleen earth is warm [and] harmonious, the middle burner is automatically treated, [managed or at peace,] the diaphragm is open, [and one] is able to eat. (脾土温和，中焦自治，膈开能食矣。 *Pi tu wen he, zhong jiao zi zhi, ge kai neng shi yi.*)
This statement also implies that yang qi or warmth is necessary for proper spleen/middle burner function and the ability to eat and digest food.

The spleen is the source of engenderment [and] transformation. (脾为生化之源 *Pi wei sheng hua zhi yuan.*)

The spleen is the viscus of transformation [and] engenderment of the qi [and] blood. (脾为化生气血之脏 *Pi wei hua zhu xie zhi zang.*)

The spleen is the root of the constructive [and] blood. (脾为营血之本 *Pi wei ying xue zhi ben.*)
These statements mean that the spleen is the source of engenderment and transformation of the qi, blood, and body fluids from the finest essence (精微, *jing wei*) of the food and drink (水谷, *shui gu*, literally water and grains).

The spleen qi scatters essence.[3] (脾气散精。 *Pi qi san jing.*)
The essence that the spleen qi scatters or disperses is the finest essence of food and drink.

The spleen governs movement [and] transformation. (脾主运化 *Pi zhu yun hua.*)

---

[3] According to Wiseman *et al.*, 散 (*san*) should be translated as dissipate. However, I prefer the word "scatter." This Chinese word also means powder. Therefore, the image is the scattering of powder when blown away.

The spleen governs the movement and transformation of food and drink and water fluids in the body.

Spleen qi vacuity leads to loss of duty of movement and transformation [with] water dampness collecting internally. (脾气虚则运化失职，水湿内停。*Pi qi xu ze yun hua shi zhi, shui shi nei ting.*)

Because the spleen governs movement and transformation, if, for any reason, the spleen qi becomes vacuous and weak, it may fail to move and transform water fluids. These stop or collect and accumulate, transforming into evil dampness internally.

[If] the spleen [and] stomach are vacuous [and] weak, [they] are not able to control [and] disperse water [and] thick liquids. Therefore, [one] has phlegm rheum. (脾胃虚弱，不能克消水浆，故有痰饮也。*Pi wei xu ruo, bu neng ke xiao shui jiang, gu you tan yin ye.*)

[If] spleen earth [is] vacuous [and] damp, the clear [has] difficulty being upborne [and] the turbid [has] difficulty being downborne. [Instead, it] flows into the center [and] stagnates [in] the diaphragm. [Thus it becomes] depressed and produces phlegm. (脾土虚湿，清者难升，浊者难降，流中滞膈，郁而成痰。*Pi tu xu shi, qing zhe nan sheng, zhuo zhe nan jiang, liu zhong zhi ge, yu er cheng tan.*)

These two statements reiterate the preceding statement *vis à vis* the spleen's control over the movement and transformation of water fluids. If dampness lingers and endures, it congeals into phlegm.

The spleen is the source of the engenderment of phlegm. (脾为生痰之源. *Pi wei sheng tan zhi yuan.*)

Because the spleen governs the movement and transformation of water fluids, if water fluids collect and transform into dampness and dampness lingers and endures, congealing into phlegm, it is said that the spleen is the source of the engenderment of phlegm.

[If] the spleen [and] stomach contract damage, water erroneously makes dampness, grains erroneously make stagnation, [and] the efflorescence of the qi is not able [to be] transported [and] transformed. (脾胃受伤则水反为湿，谷反为滞，精华之气，不能输化。 *Pi wei shou shang ze shui fan wei shi, gu fan wei zhi, jing hua zhi qi, bu neng shu hua.*)

If the spleen and stomach are damaged, not only may dampness accumulate but food stagnation may also be engendered, nor will the rest of the body obtain its supplies for construction and nourishment.

The spleen manages the blood. (脾统血 *Pi tong xue.*)

This means that it is the spleen qi which contains or holds the blood within its vessels.

Spleen yang vacuity leads to inability to gather [or contain] the blood. (脾阳虚，则不能统血。 *Pi yang xu, ze bu neng tong xue.*)

As a corollary of the preceding statement, if the spleen yang qi becomes vacuous and weak, it may fail to contain the blood within its vessels, thus resulting in various hemorrhagic conditions.

The spleen stores the constructive. (脾藏营 *Pi cang ying.*)

The constructive refers to the constructive qi which is derived from the finest essence of food and drink.

The spleen governs the muscles [and] flesh. (脾主肌肉 *Pi zhu ji rou.*)

This means that the spleen governs both the shape and the strength of the muscles and flesh. This is an extension of the spleen's being the latter heaven root of the engenderment and transformation of qi and blood. It is the qi which empowers or gives strength to the muscles and the blood which nourishes the muscles and flesh.

The spleen governs the four limbs. (脾主四肢 *Pi zhu si zhi.*)

This statement is an extension of the above. The spleen governs the muscles and flesh of the four limbs.

Spleen qi vacuity leads to nonuse of the four limbs. (脾气虚则四肢不用。 *Pi qi xu ze si zhi bu yong.*)

If the spleen qi is vacuous and weak, there is no strength (力, *lì*) to empower the function (用, *yong*) of the four limbs. In clinical practice, lack or loss of strength typically indicates a spleen qi vacuity weakness.

[If] the spleen [and] stomach are fortified, the four limbs obtain endowment of grain qi, the vessels and passageways flow and move [and are] automatically able to fill the skin and warm the flesh. (脾胃健，四肢得禀谷气，脉道流行，自能充肤热肉。 *Pi wei jian, si zhi de bing gu qi, mai dao liu xing, si neng chong fu re rou.*)

The four limbs are all endowed with qi by the stomach. [If] the spleen is not able [to make] the stomach move its fluids and humors, the vessel passageways [will become] inhibited, [and] the sinews and bones, muscles and flesh will all lack the qi to engender [them]. Therefore, [they] cannot function. (四肢皆禀 气于胃，脾不能胃行其津液，脉道不利，筋骨肌肉皆无气以 生，故不用焉。 *Si zhi jie bing qi yu wei, pi bu neng wei xing qi jin ye, mai dao bu li, jin gu ji rou jie wu qi yi sheng, gu bu yong yan.*)

These are yet two more statements expressing the spleen and stomach's vital role in the construction and nourishment of the entire body.

The spleen governs the movement of stomach fluids [and] humors.[4] (脾主为胃行其津液 *Pi zhu wei wei xing qi jin ye.*)

As do all the bowels, the stomach receives its qi from its paired yin viscus, in this case the spleen. Therefore, the qi which empowers the stomach's downbearing and movement of fluids and humors ultimately comes from the spleen.

The spleen governs the latter heaven. (脾主后天 *Pi zhu hou tian.*)

---

[4] According to Wiseman *et al.*, 津液 (*jin ye*) should be translated as liquid and humor. However, I prefer "fluids" to "liquid" and I also prefer that these two words be used in the plural. Otherwise, I think the English sounds extremely stilted and strange.

The spleen is the root of latter heaven. (脾为后天之本 *Pi wei hou tian zhi ben.*)

Within Chinese medicine, the latter heaven refers to all righteous qi derived from the transformation of food and drink. Since the spleen governs this process, the spleen governs the latter heaven.

Spleen qi governs upbearing. (脾气主升 *Pi qi zhu sheng.*)

The spleen governs the upbearing of the clear (清, *qing*) part of food and drink.

The spleen governs upbearing of the clear. (脾主升清 *Pi zhu sheng qing.*)

This statement specifies exactly what the spleen is in charge of upbearing.

The spleen upbears the clear [and] transports [this] upward [to] the heart and lungs [which] scatter [and] spread the constructive [and] nourishment around the body. (脾升清，上输心肺，散布营养周身。*Pi sheng qing, shang shu xin fei, san bu ying yang zhou shen.*)

This statement makes it even clearer how the finest essence of the food and drink are upborne to the heart and lungs in order to then be circulated to the rest of the body.

The spleen appropriately upbearing leads to [its] fortification; the stomach appropriately downbearing leads to [its] harmony. (脾宣升则健，胃宣降则和。*Pi xuan sheng ze jian, wei xuan jiang ze he.*)

"Fortification" is typically the verb used to describe the supplementation of the spleen qi. "Harmony" in relationship to the stomach implies the harmonious downbearing of the stomach qi. When the stomach is disharmonious (不和, *bu he*), it means that the stomach qi is counterflowing upward (上逆, *shang ni*).

The spleen governs center earth. (脾主中土 *Pi zhu zhong tu.*)

The spleen governs the center or middle burner and corresponds to the earth phase. Therefore, the spleen governs center earth.

The spleen governs the central prefecture [or region]. (脾主中州 *Pi zhu zhong zhou.*)

The middle burner is sometimes also called the central prefecture.

The spleen is the root of the central qi. (脾为中气本 *Pi wei zhong qi ben.*)

The spleen and stomach are the two main organs in the middle burner, and it is the spleen which engenders and transforms the qi for both. Therefore, the spleen is the root of the central qi.

The spleen rules the mouth. (脾主口。*Pi zhu kou.*)

The spleen opens into the orifice of the mouth. (脾开窍于口 *Pi kai qiao yu kou.*)

These two statements mean that, according to five phase theory, the mouth corresponds to the spleen, and diseases of the mouth may reflect disorders of the spleen.

The spleen pulse is moderate. (脾脉缓 *Pi mai huan.*)

The moderate pulse can either be a healthy, normal pulse or a diseased pulse. Here it means a healthy, normal pulse. That means it is neither too big or too small, neither floating or deep, not overly slippery and not bowstring or wiry.

The spleen has its efflorescence in the four whites of the eyes. (脾其华在眼四白 *Pi qi hua zai yan si bai.*)

According to five phase theory, the part of the eyes that corresponds to the spleen are the four whites.

Spleen qi flows freely to [or connects with] the mouth. (脾气通于口 *Pi qi tong yu kou.*)

This statement reiterates the connection between the spleen and the mouth.

The spleen stores reflection. (脾藏意 *Pi cang yi.*)

Thought is the orientation [*i.e.,* emotion] of the spleen. (脾志为思 *Pi zhi wei si.*)

The ability to think and reflect corresponds to the spleen. Therefore, excessive thinking, as in worry, damages the spleen and can also be an indication that the spleen has been damaged.

The spleen forms drool. (脾为涎 *Pi wei xian.*)

Drool is the humor of the spleen. (涎为脾液 *Xian wei pi ye.*)

Drool is one of the five humors according to five phase theory. Drool springs from the cheeks and flows from the corners of the mouth during sleep. As these two statements make clear, drool is the humor that corresponds to the spleen.

The spleen is averse to dampness. (脾恶湿 *Pi wu shi.*)

This means that either externally contracted or internally engendered dampness may damage the spleen.

The spleen rules the qi of the five viscera. (脾主五脏之气 *Pi zhu wu zang zhi qi.*)

The spleen rules the qi of the five viscera because the spleen is the latter heaven root of the engenderment and transformation of qi of the entire body.

The spleen is effulgent in the four seasons. (脾旺四时 *Pi wang si shi.*)

According to one point of view within five phase theory, the spleen should be healthy and strong throughout the year independent of the changes in seasons.

The spleen governs long summer. (脾主长夏 *Pi zhu chang xia.*)

The spleen is earth,... king of the four seasons [but] especially king of long summer. (脾者土也，... 王于四季，正王长夏。 *Pi zhe tu ye,... wang yu si ji, zheng wang chang xia.*)

However, from another point of view within five phase theory, the spleen in particular governs what Chinese call long summer. In American English, long summer is called Indian summer. It is the transition between summer and fall. In point of fact, this is a time when the spleen is easily damaged by eating too many uncooked and cool and cold natured fruits and vegetables which come ripe this time of year.

The corresponding qi of long summer nourishes the spleen. (应长夏之气以养脾。 *Ying chang xia zhi qi yi yang pi.*)

> If the weather of long summer is warm and relatively dry, this can benefit the spleen according to five phase theory as can the abundance of food at this time of year. In underdeveloped agrarian societies where famine is a real concern, long summer is typically a time of good nutrition.

[If] the spleen [is] effulgent [in] the four seasons, [there is] no contraction of evils. (四季脾旺不受邪。 *Si ji pi wang bu shou xie.*)

> In other words, if the spleen qi is effulgent throughout the year, righteous qi is adequately engendered internally and evil qi cannot enter and assail.

The large [*i.e.,* upper] abdomen governs the spleen. (大腹主脾 *Da fu zhu pi.*)

> The spleen is anatomically located in the upper abdomen.

The color yellow pertains to the spleen. (黄色属脾 *Huang se shu pi.*)

> According to five phase theory, the spleen corresponds to the earth phase and, therefore, the color yellow. In clinical practice, a yellow-colored facial complexion often indicates spleen disease.

The sweet flavor enters the spleen. (甘为入脾 *Gan wei ru pi.*)

> Similar to the above, the sweet flavor corresponds to the spleen via the earth phase. The sweet flavor in small, naturally occurring amounts supplements the spleen qi, but in excessive amounts damages the spleen by engendering dampness.

The spleen [and] stomach are the officials of the granary. (脾胃 为仓廪之官 *Pi wei wei cang lin zhi guan.*)

> According to the *Nei Jing (Inner Classic)*'s schema of the 12 officials, the spleen and stomach are the officials of the granary because these two organs are responsible for the supplies of qi and blood to construct and nourish the entire body.

The spleen is united with the stomach. (脾合胃 *Pi he wei.*)

The spleen [and] stomach [stand in] a mutual interior-exterior [relationship]. (脾与胃相表里 *Pi yu wei xiang biao li.*)

As these two statements make clear, the spleen and stomach have a yin-yang, interior-exterior relationship, and their function is interdependent.

The two qi of the spleen [and] stomach together make up the exterior [and] the interior. The stomach receives grains and the spleen rottens them. [If these] two qi are level [and] regulated, grain is transformed and [one] can eat. (脾胃二气相为表里，胃受谷而脾腐之，二气平调，则谷化而能食。*Pi wei er qi xiang wei biao li, wei shou gu er pi fu zhi, er qi ping tiao, ze gu hua er neng shi.*)

The stomach commands reception [and] absorption, [while] the spleen governs movement [and] transformation. One moves [and] one absorbs, [together] transforming [and] engendering the essence [and] qi. (胃司受纳，脾主运化，一运一纳，化生精气。*Wei si shou na, pi zhu yun hua, yi yun yi na, hua sheng jing qi.*)

These two statements clarify the respective functions of the spleen and stomach when working harmoniously as a pair.

Spleen yang is rooted in kidney yang. (脾阳根于肾阳。*Pi yang gen yu shen yang.*)

The former and latter heavens are mutually rooted. However, in particular, spleen yang is rooted in kidney yang. That means, if kidney yang declines and becomes debilitated, spleen yang qi will also become vacuous and weak and vice versa. This relationship between the spleen qi and kidney yang is an especially important one in clinical practice.

[If] tai yin damp earth obtains yang, only then [can it] move. [If] yang ming dry earth obtains yin, [it is] automatically quiet. (太阴湿土，得阳始运，阳明燥土，得阴自安。*Tai yin shi tu, de yang shi yun, yang ming zao tu, de yin zi an.*)

According to this statement, the spleen requires yang qi in order for it to perform its functions of moving and transformation. On the other hand, the stomach must obtain sufficient yin fluids to nourish and moisten it in order for its qi to harmoniously downbear and not upbear.

Internal damage [of] the spleen [and] stomach causes engenderment [of] hundreds [of] diseases. (内伤脾胃，百病由生。*Nei shang pi wei, bai bing you sheng.*)
> Because the spleen and stomach are the latter heaven source of qi and blood for the entire body, if they are damaged, this may give rise to all sorts of disease conditions and may play a part in many complicated disease mechanisms.

[If] the earth qi is full [and] harmonious, then the liver follows the spleen's upbearing [and] the gallbladder follows the stomach's downbearing. (土气充和则肝随脾升, 胆随胃降。*Tu qi chong he ze gan sui pi sheng, dan sui wei jiang.*)
> This statement implies that if the spleen qi is full and the stomach qi is harmonious, liver-gallbladder function will also tend to be normal.

Stomach
(胃, *wei*)

The stomach governs intake. (胃主受纳　*Wei zhu shou na.*)
> This means that the stomach governs the intake of food and drink.

The stomach rules the intake of grains. (胃主纳谷　*Wei zhu na gu.*)
> In this statement, "grains" stands for all foods. It is a reiteration of the preceding statement.

The stomach is the sea of water [and] grains; [it has] lots of qi and lots of blood. (胃为水谷之海，多气多血　*Wei wei shui gu zhi hai, duo qi duo xue.*)
> Because food and drink first accumulate in the stomach, it is called the sea of water and grains. Because the stomach is a very active organ and is directly supplied with qi by the spleen, it is said to have lots of qi and lots of blood.

The place from which humans receive qi is grain. The place where grain pours into is the stomach. [Therefore,] the stomach is the sea of water [and] grain, qi [and] blood. (人之所受气者，谷也. 谷之所注者，胃也。胃者，水谷气血之海也。 *Ren zhi suo shou qi zhe, gu ye. Gu zhi suo zhu zhe, wei ye. Wei zhe, shui gu qi xue zhi hai ye.*)

This statement further reiterates the above.

Water [and] grains enter the stomach [which] engenders [and] transforms fluids [and] humors. (水谷入胃，化生津液 *Shui gu ru wei, hua sheng jin ye.*)

While the stomach receives both food and drink, the stomach qi is what sends the water fluids downward to the small and large intestines to become the fluids and humors. The more active the stomach is, the more fluids it sends downwards.

[When] water [and] grains enter the mouth, the stomach is replete and the intestines are vacuous. [When] food descends, the intestines are replete and the stomach is vacuous. (水谷入口，则胃实而肠虚，食下，则肠实而胃虚。 *Shui gu ru kou, ze wei shi er chang xu, shi xia, ze chang shi er wei xu.*)

This is simply an anatomical observation. When the food enters the stomach, the stomach is relatively full and the intestines are relatively empty. When the digestate exits the stomach and enters the intestines, the intestines are relatively full and the stomach is relatively empty.

The stomach governs downbearing of the turbid. (胃主降浊 *Wei zhu jiang zhou.*)

It is the stomach qi which downbears the turbid part of food and drink to the intestines.

The stomach governs decomposition. (胃主腐熟 *Wei zhu fu shu.*)

"Decomposition" is literally "rottening and ripening." The stomach is like a fermentation tun and the food and drink in it are like a fermenting or decomposing mash.

The stomach governs free flow [and] downbearing. (胃主通降。 *Wei zhu tong jiang.*)

This means that the stomach governs the free flow and downbearing of the turbid part of food and drink to the intestines.

The mouth qi communicates with [or flows freely to] the stomach. (口气通于胃 *Kou qi tong yu wei.*)

> Previously, we saw that the mouth connected with the spleen. However, it can also be said that the mouth connects with the stomach. Therefore, problems with the mouth can indicate either spleen or stomach disorders.

The four limbs are endowed with qi from the stomach. (四肢禀气于胃 *Si zhi bing qi yu wei.*)

> Also previously, we saw that the four limbs are endowed with qi and blood by the spleen. However, the spleen and stomach work in complete interdependence, and sometimes the stomach is spoken of instead of the spleen. In that case, one should not be doctrinaire and think that only the stomach is being spoken of. Rather, the stomach is serving as a trope for the spleen-stomach or middle burner as a unit.

The stomach is yang earth. (胃为阳土 *Wei wei yang tu.*)

> If the spleen is yin earth, the stomach is yang earth.

The stomach likes harmony and downbearing. (胃喜和降 *Wei xi he jiang.*)

> As we have seen above, stomach harmony *ipso facto* means the downward movement of the stomach qi. This is the stomach qi's natural, healthy direction of movement.

The stomach governs free flow [and] downbearing. (胃主通降。 *Wei zhu tong jiang.*)

> It is said that the bowels function when they are freely flowing. This statement therefore means that the free flow and the downbearing of the small and large intestines are governed or affected by the free flow and downbearing of the stomach qi.

The stomach is the origin of the defensive qi. (胃乃卫气源 *Wei nai wei qi yuan.*)

> Again, here the stomach is being used as a trope for the spleen-stomach. The defensive qi exits from the middle burner as part of the finest essence of food and drink.

Drink and food enter the stomach [where] essence qi swims about and overflows; [these] are transported upward to the spleen. (饮食入胃，游溢精气，上输于脾 *Yin shi ru wei, you yi jing qi, shang shu yu pi.*)

> The essence qi spoken of in this statement is the finest essence of food and drink. This statement explains that this finest essence is transported upward to the spleen.

The stomach is the elder of the 12 channels. (胃为十二经之长 *Wei wei shi er jing zhi chang.*)

> If it were not for the stomach's intake of food and drink, there would be no qi and blood to flow through the channels and network vessels. Therefore, the stomach is the elder of the 12 channels.

Because stomach qi is the root of humans, if there is stomach, there is life. (人以胃气为本　有胃则生 *Ren yi wei qi wei ben, you wei ze sheng.*)

Having stomach qi leads to life; without stomach qi, there is death. (有胃气则生，无胃气则死。*You wei qi ze sheng, wu wei qi ze si.*)

> If the stomach is not able to initiate the process of digestion (消化, *xiao hua*, literally dispersion and transformation), there is no engenderment of righteous qi, and without qi, there is no life. Thus the inability to eat is considered an ominous development in a seriously ill person.

The five viscera and six bowels are all endowed with qi from the stomach; if stomach qi is effulgent, the five viscera receive their boons. (五脏六腑皆禀气于胃，胃气旺则五脏受荫 *Wu zang liu fu jie bing qi yu wei, wei qi wang ze wu zang shou yin.*)

The stomach is the sea of the five viscera [and] six bowels whose clear qi ascends to pour into the lungs. (胃为五脏六府之海，其清气上注于肺。*Wei wei wu zang liu fu zhi hai, qi qing qi shang zhu yu fei.*)

> Once again, the stomach is being used as a trope for the spleen-stomach. However, in the second statement, it says that the clear qi

upborne by the spleen-stomach pours into the lungs. It is then from the lungs that the qi is diffused and downborne to the rest of the body.

The stomach qi ascends [and] pours into the lungs. (胃气上注于肺。 *Wei qi shang zhu yu fei.*)

It is the clear qi which ascends to pour into the lungs, not specifically the stomach qi. Here the stomach qi is being used as a trope for the clear qi upborne by the spleen.

The stomach governs the moistening of the ancestral sinews, the tying of the bones, and the disinhibiting of the joints. (胃主润宗筋而束骨利关节 *Wei zhu run zong jin er shu gu li guan jie.*)

Because the stomach initiates the process of the engenderment and transformation of fluids and humors and the sinews, bones, and joints can only function if they are properly lubricated, it is said that the stomach governs the moistening of the ancestral sinews, the tying of the bones, and the disinhibiting of the joints.

If stomach middle and source qi are exuberant, one can eat and not be damaged and go beyond [meal] times and not be hungry. (胃中元气盛，则能食而不伤，过时而不饥 *Wei zhong yuan qi sheng, ze neng shi er bu shang, guo shi er bu ji.*)

If the stomach and middle burner qi are exuberant, the stomach can take in lots of food and not be damaged by food stagnation. The source qi here refers to the latter heaven source qi, the constructive qi (营气, *ying qi*). If the constructive qi is exuberant, one can go for some time and still not be hungry or run out of energy.

[If] the spleen [and] stomach are at ease [and] effulgent, [one] can eat and [become] fat. (脾胃镇旺，则能食而肥 *Pi wei zhen wang, ze neng shi er fei.*)

In premodern China, starvation was a real issue, and being fat was a positive thing (at least up to a point). It meant that one had plenty of food. If the spleen and stomach are healthy and strong or effulgent, then the person can eat a lot of food and the nutritive value of this food can be stored as fat. That being said, in the last 20 years, fat has taken on a pejorative connotation in China where there is currently an epidemic of obesity similar to that in developed Western countries.

The stomach is the central pivot [for] the upbearing [and] down-bearing of yin and yang. (胃为中枢，升降阴阳 *Wei wei zhong shu, sheng jiang yin yang.*)

In point of fact, it is the middle burner or the spleen and stomach which is the pivot for the upbearing and downbearing of yin and yang within the body.

The stomach rules the assembly of the six bowels. (胃主六腑总司 *Wei zhu liu fu zong si.*)

All six bowels have to do with the movement and eventual discharge of the turbid part of food and drink within the body. Since this process begins in the stomach, the stomach rules the assembly of the six bowels.

All the qi [and] flavor of the five viscera [and] six bowels exit from the stomach, [and] their changes are seen in the qi mouth. (五脏六腑之气味皆出于胃，变见于气口 *Wu zang liu fu zhi qi wei jie chu yu wei, bian jian yu qi kou.*)

Qi and flavor are two parts of every food. Qi is the relatively clear part which engenders yang function, while flavor is the relatively turbid part which is transformed into yin form or substance. All the qi and flavor of food must exit from the stomach before anything else can happen to it. In addition, the complete exiting of the qi and flavor of food is reflected in the tongue fur. If the qi and flavor of food exits the stomach properly, the tongue fur is thin and clear. If the qi and flavor are retained in the stomach, the tongue fur is thick and turbid.

The five flavors enter the mouth and are treasured in the intestines [and] stomach; if these flavors are treasured there, thus the five qi are nourished. (五味入口，藏于肠胃，味有所藏，以养五气 *Wu wei ru kou, cang yu chang wei, wei you suo cang, yi yang wu qi.*)

Here we are told that the five flavors nourish the qi and we are talking about food. In Chinese medicine, the word "nourish" (养, yang) always refers to yin, blood, and fluids. Therefore, if the five flavors are transformed or reabsorbed by the intestines and stomach, they become the fluids and humors, and the yin fluids and humors are then able to nourish the yang qi.

The large intestine [and] small intestine both home to the stomach. (大肠小肠皆属于胃。 *Da chang xiao chang jie shu yu wei.*)

> This means that the small intestine is connected to the stomach and the large intestine is connected to the small intestine. Therefore, whatever is going on in the stomach tends to affect the small and large intestines.

Lungs
(肺, *fei*)

The lungs pertain to metal. (肺属金 *Fei shu jin.*)

> According to five phase theory, the lungs correspond to the metal phase.

Heaven's qi flows freely to [or communicates with] the lungs. (天气通于肺。 *Tian qi tong yu fei.*)

> "Heaven's qi" refers to the great qi or atmospheric qi, the qi that we breathe in. The lungs are the organ of respiration. Therefore, heaven's qi flows free to the lungs.

The lungs govern the qi. (肺主气 *Fei zhu qi.*)

The lungs govern the qi of the entire body. (肺主一身之气 *Fei zhu yi shen zhi qi.*)

The lungs are the root of qi; all qi entirely homes to the lungs. (肺者气之本，诸气者皆属于肺 *Fei zhe qi zhi ben, zhu qi zhe jie shu yu fei.*)

> All three of these statements say that the lungs govern the qi. This means that the lungs participate in the engenderment and transformation of the qi. The clear qi upborne by the spleen combines with the great qi (大气, *da qi*) inhaled by the lungs and essence sent up by the kidneys. It also means that the lungs govern the diffusion of the qi throughout the entire body.

The chest center [or *dan zhong*] is the sea of qi. (膻中者气之海 *Dan zhong zhe qi zhi hai.*)

Above, we saw that the *dan zhong* was equated with the heart ruler or pericardium. Here, the dan zhong is equated with the lungs and thorax as the sea of qi.

The chest center [or *dan zhong*] is the sea of the ancestral [or gathered] qi. (膻中者，宗气之海。 *Dan zhong zhe, zong qi zhi hai.*)

This statement makes the meaning of the foregoing statement explicit. The *dan zhong* is the chest wherein the ancestral qi is located.

The lung qi assists the heart to move the blood. (肺气助心行血。 *Fei qi zhu xin xing xue.*)

This statement explicitly says that the lung qi aids the heart qi in the movement of the blood. As stated above, together, the heart and lung qi make up the ancestral or gathered qi.

The lungs are the governor of qi; the kidneys are the root of qi. (肺为气之主， 肾为气主根 *Fei wei qi zhi zhu, shen wei qi zhu gen.*)

The lungs are the governor of qi because it is the lung qi which empowers the diffusion and movement of the constructive and defensive qi throughout the body. However, the kidneys are the root of qi because some kidney essence is required in order to engender and transform the constructive and defensive qi.

The lungs govern the skin [and] hair. (肺主皮毛 *Fei zhu pi mao.*)

Here the hair referred to is the body hair, not the hair on the top of the head. According to five phase theory, the lungs and skin both correspond to the metal phase. Therefore, the lungs govern the skin and hair. In clinical practice, dermatological conditions are often associated with the lungs. The term "skin and hair" in most instances is simply a figure of speech for skin, remembering that the Chinese like to use two syllable constructions.

The lungs govern the voice. (肺主声 *Fei zhu sheng.*)

The voice is produced by the exhalation of air from the lungs. Therefore, the lungs govern the strength and timbre of the voice. They do not, however, govern the speech.

The lungs govern depurative downbearing. (肺主肃降 *Fei zhu su jiang.*)

Depurative downbearing or depuration and downbearing refer to the lung qi's downward diffusion of both the qi and fluids throughout the rest of the body.

The lungs are the viscus of clearing [and] depurating. (肺为清肃之脏 *Fei wei qing su zhi zang.*)

The lungs rid the stale air from the body. They also send fluids downward so they do not accumulate in the lungs and congeal into phlegm. Thus the lungs clear and depurate.

The lungs govern diffusion [and] effusion. (肺主宣发 *Fei zhu xuan fa.*)

The lungs like diffusing [and] discharging. (肺喜宣泄 *Fei xi xuan xie.*)

The lungs function normally and healthily when they are diffusing and discharging, but their function is hindered and obstructed when this diffusion and discharge are hindered and obstructed.

Diffusion means to scatter the qi and fluids throughout the body. Effusion means the effusion of the qi and sweat from the pores on the exterior of the body as well as out-thrusting (透, *tou*) any externally contracted evils that may have entered and lodged in the defensive exterior (卫表, *wai biao*).

The lungs govern the downbearing of qi. (肺主降气 *Fei zhu jiang qi.*)

The lungs govern the downbearing of the constructive and defensive qi through their diffusion and downbearing.

The lungs are the ruler of the axis of qi, [while] the spleen is the source of engenderment of the qi. (肺为主气之枢，脾为生气之源。 *Fei wei zhu qi zhi shu, pi wei sheng qi zhi yuan.*)

The axis or pivot of qi implies the qi mechanism or dynamic and the four movements of the qi—upbearing, downbearing, entering, and exiting. The lungs via respiration govern these four movements of the qi. However, it is the spleen which engenders the qi.

The lungs govern order [and] discipline. (肺主治节 *Fei zhu zhi jie.*)

Breathing is a process of inhalation followed by exhalation always repeated in an orderly and disciplined or divided way and the lungs govern respiration.

The lungs depend on nourishment from the spleen. (肺寄养于脾 *Fei ji yang yu pi.*)

The lung qi is upborne by the spleen. Therefore, if the spleen qi becomes vacuous and weak, the lung qi may become vacuous and insufficient.

Downbearing on the right of a person's body pertains to the lungs. (人身右降属肺 *Ren shen you jiang shu fei.*)

We have seen above how upbearing on the left pertains to the liver. Here, downbearing on the right pertains to the lungs. However, this is a theoretic yin-yang dichotomy which is little if ever used in clinical practice today.

The lungs govern the movement of water. (肺主行水 *Fei zhu xing shui.*)

The lungs govern the free flow [and] regulation of the waterways. (肺主通调水道 *Fei zhu tong tiao shui dao.*)

The lungs diffuse and downbear water fluids in the body. Therefore, it is said that the lungs govern the free flow and regulation of the waterways.

The lungs are the upper source of water. (肺为水之上源 *Fei wie shui zhi shang yuan.*)

In Chinese medicine, the three viscera which control the movement and transformation of water fluids in the body are the lungs, spleen, and kidneys, and each one of these resides in one of the three burners, upper, middle, and lower respectively. Therefore, the lungs are the upper source of water.

The lungs govern the transportation of essence to the skin [and] hair. (肺主输精于皮毛 *Fei zhu shu jing yu pi mao.*)

It is primarily the lung qi which moves and transports the blood and fluids to nourish and moisten the skin and hair. Here, "essence" is used as a figure of speech for blood and fluids.

The lungs govern the exterior of the entire body. (肺主一身之表 *Fei zhu yi shen zhi biao.*)

The lungs govern the defensive exterior. (肺主卫表 *Fei zhu wei biao.*)

The lungs govern both the exterior of the body and defensive qi. Therefore, the lungs govern the defensive exterior.

The lungs face the hundreds of vessels. (肺朝百脉 *Fei chao bai mai.*)

This means that all the channels and vessels in the body connect with the lungs.

The lungs are the florid canopy. (肺为華盖 *Fei wei hua gai.*)

This means the lungs are like a tent which covers all the other viscera and bowels. This has two clinical implications. First, the lungs are the first viscus usually attacked by externally invading evils. Secondly, since all heat tends to float upward, heat evils tend to accumulate in the lungs.

The lungs are the delicate viscus. (肺为娇脏 *Fei wei jiao zang.*)

This means that the lungs are easily invaded by external evils.

The lungs form snivel. (肺为涕 *Fei wei ti.*)

Snivel is the lung humor. (涕为肺之液 *Ti wei fei zhi ti.*)

According to the five phase theory, snivel or nasal mucus is the humor corresponding to the lungs. As long as the lungs are diffusing and downbearing water fluids correctly, snivel is not much seen. However, if the lungs lose their depurative downbearing, fluids collect and spill over, forming snivel.

The corresponding cool qi of fall nourishes the lungs. (应秋凉之气以养肺。 *Ying qiu liang zhi qi yi yang fei.*)

According to five phase theory, the fall season and the lungs both correspond to the metal phase. Therefore, fall is the season that corresponds to the lungs. The lung qi is often damaged by the hot, dry baking weather of late summer, and the cool weather of fall can put an end to this and benefit the lungs.

The lungs are averse to cold. (肺恶寒 *Fei wu han.*)

The lungs hold the office of assistant, and management emanates from here. (肺者相傅之关也，治節出焉 *Fei zhe xiang fu zhi guan ye, zhi jie chu yan.*)
The lungs are involved in the proper function of a number of other viscera and bowels in the body, including the spleen, kidneys, heart, and liver, large intestine, bladder, and triple burner. Therefore, the lungs act as an assistant to many other viscera and bowels. Further, by treating the lungs, we can manage a number of disorders of these other organs.

The lungs govern administering the sections. (肺主治节。 *Fei zhu zhi jie.*)
This means that the lungs govern the coordinated activities of the viscera and bowels.

The lungs are united with the skin [and] hair. (肺合皮毛 *Fei he pi mao.*)
According to five phase theory, the skin and hair as a unit are the bodily tissue corresponding to the lungs.

The lungs' efflorescence [is] in the [body] hair. (肺其华在毛 *Fei qi hua zai mao.*)
If the lungs are healthy, the body hair should likewise be healthy. As we have seen above, a number of dermatological conditions are associated with the lungs in Chinese medicine, and some dermatological conditions result in hair loss of the body.

The lung pulse is floating. (肺脉浮 *Fei mai fu.*)
The inch pulse on the right hand is sometimes referred to as the lung pulse, and it is normal for this pulse to be somewhat floating compared to the other pulse positions. When this pulse is even more obviously floating, it may indicate external contraction of evils affecting the defensive exterior and the lungs.

The lungs store the corporeal soul. (肺藏魄 *Fei cang po.*)
Under the liver above, we discussed the ethereal and corporeal
souls. The corporeal soul is associated with the animal vitality of the
individual and is said to be stored in the lungs. However, contemporary Chinese medicine makes little if any use of this concept.

Sorrow is the orientation [*i.e.*, affect or emotion] of the lungs.
(肺志为悲 *Fei zhi wei bei.*)
According to five phase theory, sorrow is the affect of the lungs. In
particular, great sorrow and grief scatter and consume the lung qi,
leading to lung qi vacuity.

The white color pertains to the lungs. (白色属肺 *Bai se shu fei.*)
According to five phase theory, the lungs and the color white both
correspond to the metal phase and, therefore, the color white
pertains to the lungs. In clinical practice, a very chalky, pale white
facial complexion may indicate a severe lung qi vacuity.

The acrid flavor enters the lungs. (辛味入肺 *Xin wei ru fei.*)
Again according to five phase theory, the acrid flavor corresponds
to the metal phase and, therefore, also to the lungs. Acrid-flavored
foods and medicinals tend to promote the diffusion of the lung qi.
Therefore, they can be used when the lung qi's diffusion is hindered
and obstructed by evils. However, overuse of acrid foods or medicinals can potentially damage and consume the lung qi.

The pharynx [and] larynx are the doors of the lungs [and]
stomach. (咽喉为肺胃之门户 *Yan hou wei fei wei zhi men hu.*)
The pharynx connects with both the esophagus and the larynx. The
esophagus connects with the stomach, and the larynx connects with
the bronchi and lungs. Therefore, the pharynx and larynx are the
doors of the lungs and stomach.

The lungs are the door of the voice. (肺为声音之门户 *Fei wei
sheng yin zhi men hu.*)
As we have seen above, exhalation from the lungs passing over the
vocal cords produces the sound of the voice. Therefore, it is no
great leap to say that the lungs are the door of the voice.

The lungs open into the orifices of the nose. (肺开窍于鼻 *Fei kai qiao yu bi.*)

> The nose is the lungs' corresponding orifice according to five phase theory. This makes sense since healthy breathing takes place mainly through the nose.

When the lungs are harmonious, the nose is able to know fragrance [from] fetor. (肺和则鼻能知香臭 *Fei he ze bi neng zhi xiang chou.*)

> Loss of smell is most often due to loss of the lungs' diffusion and downbearing. Instead, phlegm rheum collects and spills over, obstructing the nose and preventing the sense of smell.

The lungs are united with the large intestine. (肺合大肠 *Fei he da chang.*)

The lungs [and] large intestine [stand in] a mutual interior-exterior [relationship]. (肺与大肠相表里 *Fei yu da chang xiang biao li.*)

> The lungs and large intestine are the yin-interior and yang-exterior organs respectively corresponding to the metal phase.

The lungs [and] kidneys mutually engender [each other]. (肺肾相生 *Fei wei xiang sheng.*)

> According to five phase theory, the lungs (the mother phase) engender the kidneys (the child phase). However, the lungs and kidneys also work together in terms of respiration. The lungs send the qi downward and the kidneys grasp or hold this qi within the body. Therefore, a lung or kidney qi vacuity may lead to its opposite. Further, the root of all yin in the body is the kidneys. Therefore, a lung yin vacuity may lead to a kidney yin vacuity and vice versa. So the engendering relationship between the lungs and kidneys is bi-directional. It works in both ways.

Large Intestine
(大肠, *da chang*)

The large intestine governs conveyance. (大肠主传导 *Da chang zhu chuan dao.*)

The large intestine governs the conveyance [and] transformation of waste. (大肠主传化糟粕 *Da chang zhu chuan hua zao po.*)

The large intestine holds the office of conveyance; transmutation and transformation exit from here. (大肠者传导之官也，变化出焉 *Da chang zhe chuan dao zhi guan ye, bian hua chu yan.*)
All these statements state that the large intestine governs the conveyance and eventual discharge of solid wastes from the process of digestion in the form of feces.

The large intestine governs fluids. (大肠主津 *Da chang zhu jin.*)
The large intestine plays a part in the reabsorption of water fluids from the digestate. As we have seen the reabsorption of water fluids by the small intestine goes to create the thick humors within the body. The reabsorption of water fluids by the large intestine goes to create the thin liquids in the body. Thus the large intestine governs fluids.

Kidneys
(肾, *shen*)

The kidneys pertain to water. (肾属水 *Shen shu shui.*)
According to five phase theory, the kidneys correspond to the water phase.

The kidneys store essence. (肾藏精 *Shen cang jing.*)
One of the main functions of the kidneys is that they store both former and latter heaven essences.

The kidneys rule water. (肾主水 *Shen zhu shui.*)

The kidneys are the water viscus; they govern fluids [and] humors. (肾为水脏，主津液 *Shen wei shui zang, zhu jin ye.*)

The kidneys govern fluids [and] humors. (肾主津液。*Shen zhu jin ye.*)

The kidneys govern the water of the entire body. (肾主一身之水 *Shen zhu yi shen zhi shui.*)

> The kidneys are not just the water viscus because they correspond to the water phase. The kidneys are also one of the three viscera in the body which move and transform water fluids. In particular, the kidneys transform urine which they send down to the bladder for excretion.

The spleen governs dampness. [If] dampness stirs, it leads to phlegm. The kidneys govern water. [If] water floods, it also makes for phlegm. (脾主湿，湿动则为痰。肾主水，水泛亦为痰。 *Pi zhu shi, shi dong ze wei tan. Shen zhu shui, shui fan yi wei tan.*)

> As we have seen above, water which collects and accumulates transforms into dampness, and dampness which endures congeals into phlegm. Because the kidneys are one of the three viscera which govern the movement and transformation of water fluids in the body, kidney disease may lead to the engenderment of dampness and, therefore, eventually phlegm.

The kidneys govern the absorption of qi. (肾主纳气 *Shen zhu na qi.*)

> The lungs send the inhaled qi down to the kidneys which grasp or absorb it.

The kidneys govern the bones. (肾主骨 *Shen zhu gu.*)

The kidneys engender the bones and marrow. (肾生骨髓 *Shen sheng gu sui.*)

> According to five phase theory, the bones correspond to the kidneys. Therefore, disorders of the bones are often associated with kidney vacuity.

The bones engender the marrow; the brain is the sea of marrow. (骨生髓，脑为髓海 *Gu sheng sui, nao wei sui hai.*)

The teeth are the surplus of the bones. (齿为骨之余 *Chi wei gu zhi yu.*)

All these sayings connect the bones, the marrow, brain, and the teeth ultimately to the kidneys, and vacuity of the kidneys may lead to disorders of any of these.

[When] the kidneys are full, the marrow is replete. (肾充则髓实 *Shen chong ze sui shi.*)

When the kidneys are full, it means the essence is full within them. However, when the essence is full, the marrow is replete. Therefore, when the kidneys are full, the marrow is replete.

The cheeks are the roots of the bones. (颧为骨之本 *Quan wei gu zhi ben.*)

This statement is not much used in contemporary Chinese medicine. It may mean something like this. When we say that a person has good bone structure, we primarily make this judgement based on their cheekbones.

The kidneys are the water viscus. If water does not overcome fire, the bones [become] dessicated and the marrow [becomes] vacuous. Therefore, [their] thickening is not allowed [which] leads to bone pain. (肾者水脏也，今水不胜火，则骨枯而髓虚，故是不任厚，发为骨痛。 *Shen zhe shui zang ye, jin shui bu sheng huo, ze gu ku er sui xu, gu shi bu ren hou, fa wei gu tong.*)

This statement implies that it is kidney yin or water which nourishes and moistens the bones. If yin is unable to control yang, the bones become dry and the marrow becomes dessicated. Therefore, there is bone pain.

The kidneys engender the bones [and] marrow; the marrow engenders the liver. (肾生骨髓，髓生肝。 *Shen sheng gu sui, sui sheng gan.*)

The kidneys store the essence, [and] the essence engenders the marrow [which] produces the liver. (肾藏精，精生髓成肝。 *Shen cang jing, jing sheng sui cheng gan.*)

These two statements reiterate the relationship between the kidneys, bones, essence, and marrow. However, they both go on to say that the marrow engenders the liver. This last idea is not currently referred to much in standard professional Chinese medicine.

The teeth are the tips of the kidneys [and] the surplus of the bones. (齿者，肾之标，骨之余也。 *Chi zhe, shen zhi biao, gu zhi yu ye.*)

The kidneys govern the bones and the teeth are the surplus of the bones.

The kidneys are in charge of the two excretions. (肾司二便 *Shen si er bian.*)

The two excretions are urination and defecation, and the kidney qi is responsible for sealing and closing the two doors (urethra and anus) which keep these excretions within the body. As an extension of this, kidney qi vacuity failing to seal and close these two doors may lead to diarrhea and/or urinary incontinence. This is what is meant by the saying that the kidneys are in charge of the two excretions.

The kidneys control the fire of the gate of life. (肾主命门之火 *Shen zhu ming men zhi huo*)

The life-gate fire is closely associated and sometimes simply identified with kidney fire or kidney yang. When it is not identified simply as kidney yang, it is called the moving qi between the kidneys. This implies that the kidneys play a role in governing this moving qi found between them.

There are two kidneys [and] both [are] not the kidney. The left is the kidney [and] the right is the life-gate. (肾两者，非皆肾也。其左者为肾，右者为命门. *Shen liang zhe, fei jie shen ye. Qi zuo zhe wei shen, you zhe wei ming men.*)

This statement specifies that the life-gate is specifically the right kidney, kidney yang or kidney fire.

The two kidneys together are named the life-gate. (两肾总号为命门。 *Liang shen zong hao wei ming men.*)

This is a somewhat different interpretation of the life-gate as the combination of both kidney yin and kidney yang.

The kidneys govern agility. (肾主技巧 *Shen zhu ji qiao.*)

Physical agility is an innate capacity typically associated with the former heaven essence, and essence is stored in the kidneys. For instance, lack of physical agility is often associated with conditions, such as Asperger's syndrome and Down's syndrome, which Chinese medicine attributes to the former heaven.

The kidneys govern opening [and] closing. (肾主开阖 *Shen zhu kai he.*)

This means that the kidney qi governs the opening and closing of the two lower yin, the anus and urethra-cum-vagina. The urethra-cum-vagina is the front yin (前阴, *qian yin*), and the anus is the rear yin (后阴, *hou yin*).

The kidney portals open into the two yin. (肾开窍于二阴 *Shen kai qiao yu er yin.*)

The kidneys have both an upper portal (the ears) and two lower portals, the anus and urethra-cum-anus as explained above.

The kidneys govern the closing of the treasuries. (食主闭藏 *Shen zhu bi zang.*)

It is the kidney qi which secures and astringes the essence by sealing and closing the two lower yin.

The kidneys govern the five fluids. (肾主五津 *Shen zhu wu jin.*)

The state of the five fluids is dependent on the water fluids within the body as a whole, and the kidneys are instrumental through urination in controlling the volume of water fluids in the body.

The kidneys govern fear. (肾主恐 *Shen zhu kong.*)

Fear is the orientation [*i.e.,* emotion or affect] of the kidneys. (肾志为恐 *Shen zhi wei kong.*)

Fear damages the kidneys. (恐伤肾 *Kong sheng shen.*)

All three of these statements relate the affect fear to the kidneys. This is a five phase correspondence. In particular, great or excessive fear damages the kidneys.

The kidneys store the will. (肾藏志 *Shen cang zhi.*)

It may seem far-fetched to relate willpower to the kidneys. However, in clinical practice, long-distance and endurance athletes typically do not show many signs or symptoms of kidney vacuity. Instead, they show signs and symptoms of spleen vacuity. So there may be some truth that one's ability to persevere is related to the kidney qi.

The kidneys hold the office of labor, [and] agility emanates from here. (肾者作强之官，技巧出焉 *Shen zhe zuo qiang zhi guan, ji qiao chu yan.*)

This statement also implies that perseverance and the ability to work long and hard are associated with the kidneys.

The kidneys govern reproduction. (肾主生殖 *Shen zhu sheng zhi.*)

In Chinese medicine, the male gonads are sometimes referred to as the external kidneys (外肾, *wai shen*). Sexual desire is a function of kidney yang, while semen and the menstrual blood are both seen as the outward expressions of kidney essence, and conception is believed to be the product of the union of these white and red essences within the uterus. Therefore, in Chinese medicine, the kidneys govern all aspects of reproduction, and reproductive disorders are mainly treated via the kidneys.

The testes are the external kidneys. (外肾，睾丸也。 *Wai shen, gao wan ye.*)

This statement equates the male gonads with the "external kidneys."

The kidneys are the root of the former heaven. (肾为先天之本 *Shen wei xian tian zhi ben.*)

The kidneys store the former heaven essence. Therefore, they are the former heaven root.

The kidneys are the root of the source qi. (肾为元气之根本 *Shen wei yuan qi zhi gen ben.*)

There are two kinds of source qi in the body—former and latter heaven source qi. The former heaven source qi is transformed from the former heaven essence stored in the kidneys. Therefore, the kidneys are the root of the source qi.

The kidneys are the viscus of water and fire; inside [them] are true yin and true yang. (肾为水火之脏，内于真阴真阳 *Shen wei shui huo zhi zang, nei yu zhen yin zhen yang.*)

It is said that, within the body, yin and yang are water and fire respectively, and the kidneys store both true yin and true yang— true yin in the left kidney and true yang in the right kidney. Therefore, the kidneys are not simply the water viscus but the viscus of fire and water.

The kidney pulse is deep. (肾脉沉 *Shen mai chen.*)

The kidney pulse typically refers to either both cubit positions or the left cubit position. However, the cubit positions are normally somewhat deep relative to the other positions. Therefore, it is said that the kidney pulse is deep. Another way of explaining this is to posit five divisions from superficial to deep at any one of the three positions (三部, *san bu*). In this case, the most superficial position corresponds to the lungs and the deepest position corresponds to the kidneys. Therefore, from this point of view as well, the kidney pulse is deep.

The kidney pulse emits [from its] source at the heel of the foot. (肾脉发元足跟 *Shen mai fa yuan zu gen.*)

In the *Nei Jing (Inner Classic)*, there is a system of nine pulses located at nine different arteries in the body. One of these pulses is the post-tibial pulse. According to this system of pulse examination, this post-tibial pulse corresponds to the kidneys.

The kidneys' efflorescence is in the hair. (肾其华在发 *Shen qi hua zai fa.*)

This refers to the hair on the head. The loss of hair associated with aging corresponds in Chinese medicine to the decline and debility of the kidneys also associated with aging.

Kidney qi communicates with [or flows freely] to the ears. (肾气通于耳 *Shen qi tong yu er.*)

The ears are the upper orifices of the kidneys. Therefore, auditory acuity and auditory disturbances typically indicate kidney disease.

The kidney vessel networks with the root of the tongue. (肾脉络舌本 *Shen mai luo she ben.*)

The kidneys are the root of the voice. (肾为声音之根 *Shen wei shu yin zhi gen.*)

The kidneys also connect with the root of the tongue via an internal pathway. In particular, kidney yin vacuity may lead to hoarseness of the voice via this pathway.

The kidneys are the root of qi. (肾为气之本 *Shen wei qi zhi ben.*)

The kidneys are the root of qi for two reasons. First, the kidneys grasp or absorb the qi sent down by the lungs. Secondly, some kidney essence is required to engender and transform qi manufactured from the combination of the finest essence of food and drink and the great qi. Without this kidney essence, latter heaven qi cannot be made. Therefore, the kidneys are the root of qi.

The kidneys form spittle. (肾为唾 *Shen wei tuo.*)

Spittle is one of the five humors according to five phase theory and one of the two fluids Chinese medicine posits within the mouth. As such, spittle is an indication of kidney yin or water. Insufficient fluids in the mouth indicate kidney yin vacuity, while excessive fluids in the mouth may indicate a kidney yang vacuity. These yin fluids associated with the kidneys arrive under the bottom of the tongue via the internal pathway connecting the kidneys with the root of the tongue described above.

The kidneys are averse to dryness. (肾恶燥 *Shen wu zao.*)

According to five phase theory, dryness damages the kidneys. However, it is not so much external dryness that damages the kidneys as internal dryness. Internal heat may damage fluids and lead to dryness. Since the yin, blood, and fluids in the body are all connected, such dryness may eventually damage kidney yin.

The corresponding storing qi of winter nourishes the kidneys. (应冬藏之气以养肾。 *Ying dong zang zhi qi yi yang shen.*)

Again according to five phase theory, the kidneys and winter both correspond to the water phase. Therefore, the kidneys correspond to the season of winter. Winter is traditionally a time of storing up, and such storing up helps to replenish the kidneys.

The kidneys are the bar of the stomach. (肾者胃为之关 *Shen zhe wei wei zhi guan.*)

The stomach downbears turbid fluids to the small and large intestines and eventually to the kidneys and urinary bladder. However, ultimately, it is the kidneys which determine how much of these fluids are excreted as urine. So the kidneys are the bar of the stomach, preventing too many fluids from flowing out from the body. A corollary of this saying is that stomach heat is one of the disease mechanisms of polyuria. In this case, a hot stomach is hyperactive and downbears too many fluids to the kidneys.

The kidneys are the bar of the stomach [which] opens into the orifices of the two yin. [They are] the place of the opening [and] closing of the two excretions. (肾为胃关，开窍于二阴，所以二便之开闭。 *Shen wei wei guan, kai qiao yu er yin, suo yi er bian zhi kai bi.*)
This statement goes on to explain the kidney qi's control over the anus and urethra-cum-vagina as explained above.

The low back is the mansion of the kidneys. (腰为肾之府 *Yao wei shen zhi fu.*)
In Chinese medicine, the low back is closely associated with the anatomical location of the kidneys, and one of the main symptoms of either kidney yin or yang vacuity is low back soreness and pain.

The upper back is reached by the pathway of the kidneys. (背及肾之道路 *Bei ji shen zhi dao lu.*)
This means that problems with the upper back may also be associated with kidney disease.

Kidney yang should be still; stillness leads to the ability to store. (肾阳宜静，静则能藏 *Shen yang yi jing, jing ze neng cang.*)
This means that kidney yang should not be hyperactive. If yang becomes hyperactive, essence will be consumed by excessive stirring or it may be lost via seminal efflux or emission.

The kidneys govern hibernation [or dormancy]. (肾主蛰 *Shen zhu zhe.*)
Because the kidneys correspond to the water phase and storage and stillness, the kidneys govern hibernation or dormancy. In particular, the winter is a good time to be still (or more still) and store up essence in order to be able to meet the demands of the rest of the year.

Kidney essence makes the pupil [of the eye]. (肾之精为瞳子 *Shen zhi jing wei tong zi.*)

The pupils of the eyes reflect the state of kidney essence according to five phase theory.

The black color pertains to the kidneys. (黑色属肾 *Hei se shu shen.*)

[If] a black color appears on the face, one knows damage has reached the kidneys. (黑色现于面，则知伤及肾 *Hei se xian yu mian, ze zhi shang ji shen.*)
According to five phase theory, the black color corresponds to the water phase and, therefore, also to the kidneys. Therefore, a black facial complexion may indicate kidney vacuity, while black-colored foods and medicinals are often said to supplement the kidneys.

The salty flavor enters the kidney. (咸味入肾 *Xian wei ru shen.*)
Also according to the five phase theory, the salty flavor corresponds to the water phase. Thus the salty flavor is said to enter the kidneys. In Chinese herbal medicine, medicinals are often fried in salt-water in order to enable them to enter the kidneys more efficiently and effectively.

The kidneys govern the essence of the five viscera. (肾主五脏之精 *Shen zhu wu zang zhi jing.*)
Essence is stored in all five viscera. However, the major portion of the essence is stored in the kidneys. Therefore, the kidneys govern the essence of the five viscera.

The kidneys are united with the bladder. (肾合膀胱 *Shen he pang guang.*)

The kidneys [and] bladder [stand in] a mutual interior-exterior [relationship]. (肾与膀胱相表里 *Shen yu pang guang xiang biao li.*)
The kidneys and bladder have a yin-yang, interior-exterior relationship wherein the kidneys are yin and interior relative to the bladder being yang and exterior. Because of this close relationship, diseases of one organ may affect the other.

The kidneys unite with the triple burner [and] the bladder. (肾合三焦膀胱。 *Shen he san jiao pang guang.*)

Because the water passageways of the triple burner are closely related to the movement of water fluids in the body and the kidneys are one of the three viscera which govern water, the kidneys are united with or connected to the triple burner.

Kidney water moistens liver wood. (肾水涵肝木 *Shen shui han gan mu.*)

Kidney water or yin is necessary to moisten and sprinkle liver wood in order for the liver to function correctly. Therefore, kidney yin vacuity may lead to liver depression qi stagnation or liver blood and yin vacuity with or without concomitant hyperactivity of liver yang, liver heat, or liver wind.

The kidneys and large intestine [share] the same abode [in] the lower burner. (肾与大肠同居下焦。 *Shen yu da chang tong ju xia jiao.*)

While this statement may simply be read as an anatomical description of the kidneys' location, it does also point out that the kidneys and large intestine do have a clinical relationship. Enduring diarrhea can lead to kidney qi vacuity, since the kidney qi controls the sealing and closing of the anus. *Vice versa*, kidney qi vacuity can also lead to diarrhea.

The kidneys [have] no repletion patterns. (肾无实证. *Shen wu shi zheng.*)

The kidneys [have] no draining methods. (肾无泻法. *Shen wu xie fa.*)

Both of these statements point to the same thing. In standard professional Chinese medicine, there are no repletion patterns of the kidneys and, therefore, the kidneys are never treated by draining.

Urinary Bladder
(膀胱, *pang guang*)

The bladder governs storage of fluids [and] humors. (膀胱主藏津液 *Pang guang zhu cang jin ye.*)

The bladder stores the fluids and humors in that it stores the urine which is the turbid part of the fluids and humors meant for excretion.

The bladder is the mansion of fluids [and] humors. (膀胱者津液之府 *Pang guang zhe jin ye zhi fu.*)
The bladder is the official of the islet prefecture, and fluids and humors are treasured herein. [If its] qi transforms [these, they] are able to be exited. (膀胱者州都之官，津液藏焉。气化则能出矣. *Pang Guang zhe zhou dou zhi guan, jin ye cang yang. Qi hua ze neng chu yi.*)
These two statements essentially reiterate the foregoing. However, the second statement adds that it is the qi transformation (气化, *qi hua*) of the bladder which ultimately exits urine from the body.

The bladder is the abductor [and] leader of water. (膀胱为水之导引 *Pang guang wei shui zhi dao yin.*)
As stated above, it is the bladder qi which abducts and leads turbid water out of the body as urine.

Triple Burner
(三焦, *san jiao*)

The triple burner has a name but no form. (三焦有名无形 *San jiao you ming wu xing.*)
This means that the triple burner or three burners are merely an abstract concept that has no individual anatomical existence.

The triple burner is one name [but] three concerns [or things]. (未三焦者，一名三关也。 *Wei san jiao zhe, yi ming san guan ye.*)

The head to the heart is the upper burner, the heart to the navel is the middle burner, [and] the navel to the feet is the lower burner. (头至心为上焦，心至脐为中焦，脐至足为下焦。 *Tou zhi xin wei shang jiao, xin zhi qi wei zhong jiao, qi zhi zu wei xia jiao.*)
These two statements convey the majority opinion in contemporary Chinese medicine. The three burners are nothing more than a

description of three arbitrary anatomical divisions of the body, and the functions of the three burners or triple burner are nothing other than the coordinated function of the organs within these three anatomical divisions.

The triple burner is the function of ministerial fire. [It] divides [and] spreads life-gate source qi. [It] rules upbearing [and] downbearing, exiting [and] entering. [It] parades between heaven and earth. [It is] the overall understanding of the qi of the five viscera [and] six bowels, the constructive [and] defensive, the channels [and] network vessels, the internal [and] external, above [and] below, left [and] right. It is the business house of the bowel of the central essence. Above, [it] governs absorption; [in] the middle, [it] governs transformation, [and] below, [it] governs exiting. (三焦为相火之用，分布命门元气，主升降出入，游行天地之间，总领五脏六腑营卫经络内外上下左右之气，号中精之腑。上主纳，中主化，下主出。*San jiao wei xiang huo zhi yong, fen bu ming men yuan qi, zhu sheng jiang chu ru, you xing tian di zhi jian, zong ling wu zang liu fu ying wei jing luo nei wai shang xia zuo you zhi qi, hao zhong jing zhi fu. Shang zhu na, zhong zhu hua, xia zhu chu.*)

According to this passage by Zhang Yuan-su, the triple burner is the function of ministerial fire which spreads the life-gate source qi. It governs the four movements of the qi—upbearing and down-bearing, entering and exiting. Further, it is the overall sum total of the collected qi of the five viscera and six bowels, the constructive and defensive, the channels and network vessels, the internal and external, above and below, and right and left of the body. It is the place of business of the bowel of the central essence. The upper burner governs absorption, *i.e.*, respiration. The middle burner governs the transformation of food and drink, while the lower burner governs the exiting of the feces and urine. In this passage, the word 领 (*ling*) literally means a neck collar. In other words, it is something which holds everything else together. In this sense, it can also be rendered as the outline or general understanding of something.

The triple burner governs the sluices. (三焦主决渎 *San jiao zhu jue du.*)

The triple burner is the official of the sluices [and] homes to the bladder. (三焦者诀渎之官，属膀胱 *San jiao zhe jue du zhi guan, shu pang guang.*)
> Both of these statements refer to the water passageways of the body which carry water fluids through the body. The turbid remainder of these water fluids eventually arrive at the bladder from which they are finally excreted as urine.

The triple burner is the source of defensive [and] constructive. (三焦营卫之源 *San jiao ying wei zhi yuan.*)
> The three burners are the source of both the constructive and defensive qi. Food enters the middle burner where its finest essence is upborne by the spleen to the upper burner. The clear of the clear goes to the lungs where it unites with the great qi to become the constructive and defensive qi, and it is the lung qi which then moves this constructive and defensive qi throughout the rest of the body. (Comparatively, the constructive qi is clearer than the defensive qi, but both are engendered from the clear of the clear.) The turbid of the clear is upborne by the spleen to the heart where it becomes the blood. The heart then pumps this blood out to the rest of the body. However, for any of this to happen, some essence stored in the kidneys in the lower burner must ascend to the heart and lungs to help make the qi and blood. Therefore, the three burners are the source of the defensive and constructive qi.

The three burners are a human's three sources of qi. (三焦者，人之三元之气也。 *San jiao zhe, ren zhi san yuan zhi qi ye.*)
> This statement is a reiteration of the preceding statement.

The three burners are the passageways [and] streets of water [and] grain. (三焦者，水谷之道路。 *San jiao zhe, shui gu zhi dao lu.*)
> Because the by-products of food and drink travel through the passageways of the three burners, the three burners are the passageways and streets of water and grain.

The three burners are the parting [and] courier of the original qi [and] govern the free flow [and] movement of the three qi [which] pass through to the five viscera [and] six bowels. (三焦者，原气之别使，主通行三气，经历五脏六腑。 *San jiao zhe, yuan qi zhi bie shi, zhu tong xing san qi, jing li wu zang liu fu.*)

This statement says that the three burners are the passageways whereby the three qi move to and through the five viscera and six bowels. These three qi are the former heaven source qi of the kidneys and the latter heaven constructive and defensive qi derived from food and drink.

The upper burner is like a mist. (上焦如雾 *Shang jiao ru wu.*)
Because the lungs and heart diffuse and scatter the qi and blood to the rest of the body, the upper burner is like a mist.

The upper burner governs intake. (上焦主纳 *Shang jiao zhu na.*)
This means that the lungs within the upper burner govern the intake of the great qi.

The middle burner is like foam. (中焦如沤 *Zhong jiao ru ou.*)
The digestate rottening and ripening within the middle burner is like a foam.

The middle burner governs transformation. (中焦主化 *Zhong jiao zhu hua.*)
The spleen and stomach within the middle burner govern the transformation of food and drink.

The lower burner is like a sluice. (下焦如渎 *Xia jiao ru du.*)
The lower burner is where turbid solids and fluids in the body finally collect for excretion from the body. Therefore, the lower burner is like a sluice.

The lower burner governs exiting. (下焦主出 *Xia jiao zhu chu.*)
As stated above, the lower burner is where feces and urine exit the body from. Therefore, the lower burner governs exiting.

[The lower burner] governs the separation of clear [and] turbid. [It] governs exiting and not entering. (主分别清浊，主出而不内。*Zhu fen bie qing zhuo, zhu chu er bu nei.*)
This statement is yet another expression of the excretory role of the lower burner within human metabolism.

The lower burner... governs liver [and] kidney diseases. (下焦。。。主肝肾病候也。*Xia jiao... zhu gan shen bing hou ye.*)

Lower means the lower burner liver [and] kidney qi. (下，谓下焦肝肾之气也。 *Xia, wei xia jiao gan shen zhi qi ye.*)

These two statements say that the liver and kidney qi are both of primary importance for the health and disease of the contents of the lower burner.

The heart-wrapper network vessels [or pericardium] and triple burner stand in an exterior-interior relationship. (心包络与三焦相表里 *Xin bao luo yu san jiao xiang biao li.*)

In terms of the 12 regular channels (十二正经, *shi er zheng jing*), the pericardium and triple burner channels have a yin-yang, interior-exterior relationship, the pericardium channel being yin and interior, and the triple burner channel being yang and relatively exterior. In standard contemporary Chinese medicine, the pericardium is seen as an extension of the heart. It functions on behalf of the heart and has no independent functions of its own. Therefore, in standard professional Chinese medicine, we speak of only five viscera and six bowels.

The Life-Gate
(命门, *ming men*)

In Chinese medicine, there are a number of different interpretations of the life-gate. Therefore, some of the statements below may contradict each other.

The life-gate is the mansion of water and fire, the residence of yin and yang, the sea of essence and qi, and the hole of life and death. (命门者水火之府，阴阳之宅，精气之海，死生之窦 *Ming men zhe shui huo zhi fu, yin yang zhi zhai, jing qi zhi hai, si sheng zhi dou.*)

According to this statement, the life-gate encompasses both kidney yin and yang and thus is the root of life.

[That which] is the life-gate is the combination of the two kidneys, and the two kidneys both home to the life-gate. (是命门总乎两肾，而两肾皆属命门。 *Shi ming men zong hu liang shen, er liang shen jie shu min men.*)

This statement further equates the life-gate with the two kidneys, yin and yang, fire and water.

The life-gate is the root of the source qi [and] is the residence of water [and] fire. (命门为元气之根，为水火之宅。 *Ming men wei yuan qi zhi gen, wei shui huo zhi zhai.*)

As seen above, the life-gate is, according to some sources, identical to the kidneys. Therefore, the source qi in this statement is the kidney qi.

The life-gate is the fire of the former heaven. (命门者，先天之火也。 *Ming men zhe, xian tian zhi huo ye.*)

However, from other points of view, the life-gate refers only to kidney yang as it warms and steams the rest of the body.

The life-gate is the root of one's nature [and] destiny. It is the sea of essence [and] blood [and] the source of engenderment [and] transformation. It is the mother of the spleen [and] stomach. (命门为性命之根，精血之海，化生之源，脾胃之母 *Ming men wei xing ming zhi gen, jing xue zhi hai, hua sheng zhi yuan, pi wei zhi mu.*)

This statement first equates the life-gate with the former heaven essence since it is the former heaven essence which determines one's nature and destiny. However, it then goes on to say that it is also the ultimate source of the engenderment and transformation of latter heaven qi and blood. This is because the life-gate is the "mother" of the spleen and stomach. This means that the yang qi of the spleen and stomach are ultimately rooted in the life-gate.

The life-gate is the sea of essence [and] blood, [while] the spleen [and] stomach are the sea of water [and] grain. Both are the root of the five viscera [and] six bowels. (命门为精血之海，脾胃为水谷之海，均为五脏六腑之本。 *Ming men wei jing xue zhi hai, pi wei wei shui gu zhi hai, jun wei wu zang liu fu zhi ben.*)

Here the life-gate is posited as the sea of essence and blood in juxtaposition to the spleen and stomach which collectively are the sea of water and grains. This statement then goes on to say that both are the root of the five viscera and six bowels. In other words, the life-gate is the former heaven root and the spleen-stomach are the latter heaven root.

[If] life-gate fire declines, [it] is not able to steam [and] rotten [*i.e.*, ferment] water [and] grain. (命门火衰，不能蒸腐水谷。 *Ming men huo shuai, bu neng zheng fu shui gu.*)

The life-gate fire is the ultimate source of yang qi or heat in the body. Because the former and latter heavens are mutually rooted, the life-gate fire is the source for the yang qi of the spleen and stomach. Hence, if life-gate fire declines, the spleen and stomach will not be able to properly move and transform food and drink.

The life-gate is the source of ministerial fire, the beginning of heaven [and] earth, the treasury of essence [and] engenderer of blood. [When it] downbears, it leads to leakage; [when it] upbears, it leads to the making of lead. [It] governs the triple burner source qi. (命门为相火之原，天地之始，藏精生血，降则为漏，升则为铅，主三焦元气。 *Ming men wei xiang huo zhi yuan, tian di zhi shi, cang jing sheng xue, jiang ze wei lou, sheng ze wei qian, zhu san jiao yuan qi.*)

According to this statement, the life-gate is the source of ministerial fire. Thus ministerial is rooted in the lower burner but connects upward to the heart. The statement goes on to say that the life-gate is also the origin of heaven and earth. Since heaven and earth in the body are fire and water respectively, this means that the life-gate is the origin of kidney yin and yang. It treasures the essence and engenders the blood, remembering that blood and essence share a common source. When it downbears, it leads to leakage. This means downward movement of life-gate fire causes the blood to move frenetically outside its vessels, thus resulting in bleeding from the vagina. When it upbears, meaning when it counterflows upward, "it makes lead." Unfortunately, we have not been able to find out what Zhang Yuan-su meant by this phrase. However, according to the last part of this statement, the life-gate also governs the source qi of the triple burner.

The life-gate is ministerial fire. (命门为相火。 *Ming men wei xiang huo.*)

This statement by Qin Bo-wei makes it even more explicit that the life-gate is the ministerial fire.

The life-gate connects with the spleen. (命门和脾。 *Ming men he pi.*)
> Although the life-gate is rooted in the lower burner, it ramifies throughout the body and connects with all the tissues and organs of the body. However, it has certain connections that are closer or more important than others.

The life-gate fire warms the spleen [and] stomach. (命门之火有暖脾胃。 *Ming men zhi huo you nuan pi wei.*)
> This is a succinct statement of the relationship between the life-gate fire and the spleen and stomach.

The office of the life-gate [in] men is to store essence [and in] women is to fasten the uterus. (命门之处，男以藏精，女以系胞。 *Ming men zhi chu, nan yi zang jing, nu yi ji bao.*)
> This statement implies that the function of the life-gate is essential to sexual function and reproduction in both men and women.

The life-gate below is attached to the right kidney... [It] ascends to become the heart wrapper [or pericardium]. (命门下寄肾右...上为心包。 *Ming men xia ji shen you... shang wei xin bao.*)
> This statement says that the life-gate is attached to the right kidney, kidney yang, but that it ascends to become the pericardium. Therefore, it posits a relationship between sovereign and ministerial fires since life-gate fire is ministerial fire.

The moving qi between the kidneys. (肾间动气, *Shen jian dong qi.*)

The place which is called the origin of the living qi is the root of the 12 channels, the moving qi between the kidneys. It is the root of the five viscera [and] six bowels, the root of the 12 channels [and] vessels, the gate of the inhalation [and] exhalation, the source of the three burners. (所谓生气之原者，谓十二经之根本也，谓肾间动气也。 此五脏六腑之本，十二经脉之根，呼吸之门，三焦之原。 *Suo wei sheng qi zhi yuan zhe, wei shi er jing zhi gen ben ye, wei shen jian dong qi ye. Ci wu zang liu fu zhi ben, shi er jing mai zhi gen, hu xi zhi men, san jiao zhi yuan.*)
> This definition of the moving qi between the kidneys is very similar to some of the definitions of the life-gate above.

The life-gate connects with the heart. (命门和心。 *Ming men he xin*.)

The heart and the life-gate are the two fires of sovereign and ministerial respectively, and these two fires are interconnected. The life-gate yang qi connects with the heart yang and the two flow freely between each other.

The life-gate connects with the kidneys. (命门和肾。 *Ming men he shen*.)

As stated above, the life-gate has a close relationship with the kidneys, essentially at the least being identical to kidney yang or kidney fire.

The life-gate connects with the triple burner. (命门和三焦。 *Ming men he san jiao*.)

The life-gate is the source of being and ground of the triple burner. The life-gate yang qi flows freely to the triple burner which then spreads the life-gate's warmth to the rest of the body.

The life-gate connects with the gallbladder. (命门和胆。 *Ming men he dan*.)

The life-gate warms and nourishes gallbladder fire. Because the life-gate is ministerial fire and the gallbladder also is said to control ministerial fire, these two have a close inter-relationship.

The life-gate connects with the governing vessel. (命门和督脉。 *Ming men he du mai*.)

The governing vessel governs all the yang qi of the body and connects, either directly or indirectly, with all 12 channels. The life-gate yang qi flows freely to connect with the governing vessel and from there flows to and through all the other channels and network vessels in the body.

The Six Extraordinary Bowels
(奇恒之府, *qi heng zhi fu*)

Besides the viscera [and] bowels, there are the extraordinary bowels. These are the brain, marrow, bones, vessels, gallbladder, [and] women's uterus. (脏腑之外尚有奇恒之府，即脑髓骨脉

胆女子包。*Zang fu zhi wai shang you qi heng zhi fu. Ji nao sui gu mai dan nu zi bao.*)

The meaning of extraordinary is that they [seem] like viscera [but are] not viscera, [they seem] like bowels [but are] not bowels. [Their] form is like a bowel, but [their] function is like a viscus. (奇恒的意义是似脏非脏，似腑非腑。形虽似腑而作用似脏。*Qi heng de yi yi shi si zang fei zang, si fu fei fu. Xing sui si fu er zuo yong si zang.*)

> According to this statement, the reason that these six bowels are called extraordinary is that they seem like a viscus but are not exactly a viscus; they seem like a bowel but are not exactly a bowel. Their form is like a bowel, but they function like a viscus.

Brain
(脑, *nao*)

The brain is the mansion of the original spirit. (脑为原神之府 *Nao wei yuan shen zhi fu.*)

The brain governs the spirit brilliance. (脑主神明。*Nao zhu shen ming.*)

> These two statements are an expression of the brain-ruling theory of consciousness in Chinese medicine introduced by Li Shi-zhen in the late Ming dynasty.

The head is the mansion of bright essence. (头者，精明之府。*Tou zhe, jing ming zhi fu.*)

> While this statement does not mention the brain *per se*, it does equate the head with essence and with brightness or brilliance. As we have seen above, "spirit brilliance" is a term describing the psyche, and below we will see that the brain is the sea of marrow made from essence. Therefore, this statement also implies that the brain is the seat of the psyche.

Peoples' memory is located within the brain. Children have a tendency to forgetfulness [because their] brains are not full. The elderly have impaired memory [because their] brains gradually [become] empty. (人之记性，皆在脑中。小儿善忘者，脑未

满也。老人健忘者，脑渐空也。*Ren zhi ji xing, jie zai nao zhong. Xiao er shan wang zhe, nao wei man ye. Lao ren jian wang zhe, nao jian kong ye.*)

The inspiration [or intelligence and] memory located in the brain are due to the drink [and] food engendering the qi [and] blood. (灵机记性在脑者，因饮食生气血。*Ling ji ji xing zai nao zhe, yin yin shi sheng qi xue.*)

These two statements are yet another expression of the brain-ruling theory of consciousness within Chinese medicine. In the latter statement, the implication is that qi and blood manufacture essence which produces marrow which fills the brain where intelligence and memory are located.

[In] humans [at] the beginning of life, first essence is produced. [Once] essence [has been] produced, the brain marrow is engendered. (人始生，先成精，精成而脑髓生。*Ren shi sheng, xian cheng jing, jing cheng er nao sui sheng.*)

This statement equates the brain with marrow. Thus the brain is sometimes referred to in Chinese medicine as the sea of marrow (髓海, *sui hai*).

All the marrow homes to the brain. (诸髓者，皆属于脑。*Zhu sui zhe, jie shu yu nao.*)

Marrow is constantly being produced from essence in the body, and the ultimate respository of marrow is the brain.

Humors pour [into] the bones and supplement the brain [and] marrow. Therefore, [they] are yin. (液注骨而补脑髓。*Ye zhu gu er bu nao sui.*)

In other words, turbid fluids pour into the bones and supplement the brain marrow, remembering that the cerebrospinal fluid and intra-articular fluids are species of humor in Chinese medicine.

[If] the sea of marrow has a surplus, [one's] spry energy [has] lots of strength. (髓海有余，则轻劲多力。*Sui hai you yu, ze qing jin duo li.*)

This statement links abundant vitality to a surplus of the sea of marrow. However, one cannot have a surplus of the sea of marrow without a surplus of qi and blood. If one has a surplus of qi and blood, then one will have lots of strength and vitality.

Uterus
(胞宫, *bao gong*, 子宫, *zi gong*, 女子胞, *nu zi bao*)

The female wrapper is the child palace. (女子之胞，子宫是也。*Nu zi zhi bao, zi gong shi ye.*)
The female wrapper is the child palace. This statement is just clarifying one of the several Chinese synonyms for the uterus.

Yin [and] yang [have] intercourse [and] a fetus therefore congeals. The place where this is stored is called the child palace. (阴阳交媾，胎孕乃凝，所藏之处，名曰子宫。*Yin yang jiao gou, tai yun nai ning, suo cang zhi chu, ming yue zi gong.*)
According to Zhang Jing-yue, when men and women have intercourse and such intercourse gives rise to the conception of a fetus, the place where the fetus is stored is called the uterus.

Qi & Blood, Fluids & Humors, Essence & Spirit
(气血津液精神, *qi xue jin ye jing shen*)

Qi & Blood
(气血, *qi xue*)

Qi unites and [one] has form. (气合而有形。*Qi he er you xing.*)
In Chinese medicine, qi is not energy in the Western scientific sense of this word. Rather it is seen as a very fine or the finest form of matter. Because it is so fine, it is normally invisible. However, when qi unites, it results in form.

Qi congeals to make humans. (气凝为人。*Qi ning wei ren.*)
This saying is an extension of the previous one. Not only does the uniting of qi make form, it also specifically makes the human form or body.

[When or where] qi gathers, there is engenderment [or life]. (气 聚则生 *Qi ju ze sheng.*)

The Chinese word for engenderment, birth, and life or living are all the same (生, *sheng*). So this statement can be read in various ways. When or where the qi gathers, there is life, or, when or where the qi gathers, there is engenderment. However, in this context, we can say that it is the presence of qi which animates and gives life to the human body.

Blood is the mother of qi. (血为气母 *Xue wei qi mu.*)

This means that blood is the substance which nourishes and fuels the qi. Yin blood also controls the yang qi and keeps it from stirring frenetically and engendering wind.

Qi governs the blood. (气主血 *Qi zhu xue.*)

Qi is the commander of blood. (气为血帅 *Qi wei xue shuai.*)

Both these statements mean that 1) the qi engenders and transforms the blood, 2) moves the blood, and 3) also contains the blood within its vessels.

The ceaseless movement of the qi is like the flow of water, like the unstoppable movement of sun [and] moon. (气之不得无行也，如水之流，如日月之行不休. *Qi zhi bu de wu xing ye, ru shui zhi liu, ru ri yue zhi xing bu xiu.*)

Movement is part of qi's inherent nature. Therefore, qi's movement is ceaseless.

[If] the qi moves, the blood moves. (气行则血行 *Qi xing ze xue xing.*)

Qi is able to move the blood. (气能行血。 *Qi neng xing xue.*)

These two statements specifically imply that it is the qi which moves the blood and that the blood only moves as long as the qi propels it. In other words, the blood cannot move by itself.

The movement of qi leads to the movement of blood. Qi stagnation leads to blood congelation. Blood congelation also leads to qi stagnation. Stagnation and non-free flow lead to pain. (气行

则血行，气滞则血凝，血凝则气亦滞，滞而不通则痛. *Qi xing ze xue xing, qi zhi ze xue ning, xue ning ze qi yi zhi, zhi er bu tong ze tong*.)

> This statement further clarifies that, because the qi moves the blood, qi stagnation may lead to blood congelation or stasis. However, because the blood is the mother of the qi, blood stasis may also lead to qi stagnation. Further, stagnation and lack of free flow of the qi and blood lead to pain.

The blood [does] not move itself. It follows the qi and therefore moves. [If] the qi is stagnant within [the blood], the blood is caused to collect [and] accumulate, congeal and not scatter. (血不自行，随气乃行。气滞于中，血因停积，凝而不散. *Xue bu zi xing, sui qi nai xing. Qi zhi yu zhong, xue yin ting ji, ning er bu san*.)

> This statement specifically says that the blood does not move itself but that the qi moves it. Like other such statements above, it then goes on to explain that unmoving blood creates blood stasis.

The hair is the surplus of the blood; the spirit is the surplus of the qi. (发为血之余，神为气之余 *Fa wei xue zhi yu, shen wei qi zhi yu*.)

> The first part of this statement says that hair is nothing other than the surplus of blood, that it is made out of blood. The second part says that spirit is nothing other than a "surplus" or accumulation of qi. In other words, spirit is qi. It is just enough qi in one place that it manifests as consciousness.

Qi has the function of engendering of the blood. (气有生血之功 *Qi you sheng xue zhi gong*.)

Qi is able to engender the blood. (气能生血。 *Qi neng sheng xue*)

> Without sufficient qi, there is no power to engender and transform the blood. Based on this statement, in clinical practice, we often combine some qi supplements with blood-supplementing medicinals to more efficiently engender the blood.

Blood is able to engender the qi. (血能生气。 *Xue neng sheng qi*.)

> Because blood is the mother of qi and is needed to engender the qi, we can also say that blood is able to engender the qi. However, this

is not a common saying since it violates the basic yin-yang dichotomy inherent in Chinese medical terminology. In general, the word "engender" is always and only used to describe the function of the yang qi.

Blood has the powers to harmonize the qi. (血有和气之力 *Xue you he qi zhi li.*)
This means that blood keeps the qi from floating upward and outward and stirring frenetically.

Blood is able to hold the qi. (血能载气。*Xue neng zai qi.*)
This statement says that blood has the ability to hold the qi in its proper place.

[If] qi does not obtain blood, it leads to scattering and lack of gathering into one. (气不得血，则散而无统。*Qi bu de xue, ze san er wu tong.*)
This statement further clarifies that a sufficiency of blood is necessary to prevent qi from scattering. This all has to do with blood being the mother of qi.

Qi gathers together the blood; blood beautifies the qi. (气所以统血，血所以俪气 *Qi suo yi tong xue, xue suo yi li qi.*)
Qi manages or contains the blood within its vessels and, therefore, within the body, while blood nourishes the qi and allows it to become exuberant and flourishing.

Qi enables the containment of blood. (气能摄血 *Qi neng she xue.*)

Qi returns the blood [to the vessels]. (气为血归 *Qi wei xue gui.*)
These are yet again statements that it is the qi which holds the blood within its vessels.

Clear qi exists above; turbid qi exists below. (清气在上，浊气在下 *Qing qi zai shang, zhuo qi zai xia.*)
The clear qi exiting above refers to consciousness connecting with the outside world via the seven clear (sense) orifices or organs located above in the head. These are the mouth, the two nostrils, the two ears, and the two eyes, *i.e.*, seven. Turbid qi exiting below

refers to the urine and feces discharged from the anus and urethra in the lower part of the body.

Lesser fire engenders the qi, [and] qi enables the engenderment of blood. (少火生气，气能生血 *Shao huo sheng qi, qi neng sheng xue.*)
"Lesser fire" refers to the life-gate/ministerial fire rooted in the lower burner. As we have seen above, the life-gate is the ultimate source of all qi in the body. It is the qi, however, which then engenders the blood.

Qi effuses [or is emitted] from the viscera. (气由脏发 *Qi you zang fa.*)
The qi is engendered and then emitted from the viscera, not the bowels.

Humans receive qi from grains. (人受气于谷。*Ren shou qi yu gu.*)
Latter heaven qi comes from the finest essence of food and drink (literally water and grains) transformed by the spleen.

The central qi ascends [and] is upborne to the lungs and makes the qi. From the lungs, [it] returns [back] down to transform into the blood. (中气上升于肺而为气，从肺回下则为血。*Zhong qi shang sheng yu fei er wei qi, cong fei hui xia ze wei xue.*)
Here, the clear qi from the finest essence of food and drink is simply referred to as the central qi. This is then upborne to the lungs to become the qi. However, the passage then goes on to say that the qi then is sent back down, presumably to the middle burner, to engender the blood.

Source qi is effused from the kidneys. (元气发于肾。*Yuan qi fa yu shen.*)
Source qi refers specifically to the kidney qi which is the ultimate motivating and transforming qi in the body. Therefore, source qi is effused or emitted from the kidneys.

[If] the source qi is full [and] sufficient, the spleen [and] stomach qi suffers no damage and later is able to enrich [and] nourish the source qi. (元气充足，皆脾胃之气所无伤，而后能滋养元

气。 *Yuan qi chong zu, jie pi wei zhi qi suo wu shang, er hou neng zi yang yuan qi.*)

Because former and latter heavens are mutually rooted and mutually support and promote each other, abundant kidney qi keeps the spleen healthy, while a healthy spleen keeps the kidneys healthy by producing sufficient qi and blood to store as latter heaven essence.

The true qi is that which is received from heaven. This plus grain qi are what fill the body. (真气者，所受于天, 与谷气并而充身者也。 *Zhen qi zhe, suo shou yu tian, yu gu qi bing er chong shen zhe ye.*)

In this statement, the true qi means the former heaven kidney qi or source qi, while the grain qi is the latter heaven qi derived from the finest essence of food and drink. Together, they fill the body.

[If] qi [and] blood [are] not harmonious, the hundreds of diseases are changed [and] transformed and engendered. (气血不和，百病乃变化而生。 *Qi xue bu he, bai bing nai bian hua er sheng.*)

From one point of view, all diseases are qi and blood diseases, since yang is nothing but a lot of qi and yin is nothing but a lot of blood (and fluids). In any case, the treatment of all diseases entails the rectification and regulation of the qi and blood by some means.

Qi [desertion] follows blood desertion. (气随血脱 *Qi sui xue tuo.*)

Because the blood is the mother of the qi, extreme pathological bleeding may be followed by extreme prostration, dizziness, spontaneous sweating, and even syncope. This is referred to as qi (desertion) following blood desertion.

Qi [desertion] follows fluid desertion. (气随液脱。 *Qi sui ye tuo.*)

Similarly, because the qi travels with fluids in the body, if fluids desert, the qi may also desert. For instance, massive diarrhea and vomiting, as in cholera, may lead to qi desertion with prostration and syncope and eventual death.

Qi binding leads to blood congealing. (气结则血凝。 *Qi jie ze xue ning.*)

Qi stagnation leads to blood stasis. (气滞则血瘀。 *Qi zhi ze xue yu.*)

Qi vacuity leads to blood desertion. (气虚则血脱。 *Qi xu ze xue tuo.*)
 Qi vacuity leads to bleeding due to the qi not containing the blood within its vessels.

Qi forcing leads to blood escaping. (气迫则血走。 *Qi po ze xue zou.*)
 Frenetic movement of the qi due to heat may also cause bleeding. In this case, the hot and, therefore, hyperactive qi forces the blood to move outside its channels.

Yang qi is the warming of the qi. (阳气者，温暖之气也。 *Yang qi zhe, wen nuan zhi qi ye.*)
 Qi is inherently warm, and warming is one of its five functions. When enough qi is located in one place within the body to feel the warmth of the qi, not just its function, this is referred to as yang qi.

Qi vacuity leads to cold. (气虚则寒 *Qi xu ze han.*)
 Because qi is inherently warm, a lack of qi results in the presence of cold.

Superabundance of qi promotes the rising of fire. (气有余便是火 *Qi you yu bian shi huo.*)
 Again, because qi is inherently warm, a lot of qi in one place may transform into heat evils or even fire.

Qi is able to engender fluids. (气能生津。 *Qi neng sheng jin.*)
 Just as qi is able to engender and transform the blood, qi is able to engender fluids.

Qi is able to move fluids, (气能行津。 *Qi neng xing jin.*)
 Similarly, qi is what moves fluids in the body.

Qi is able to contain fluids. (气能摄津。 *Qi neng she jin.*)
 Further, qi is able to hold fluids within the body just as it is able to contain blood within its vessels.

Qi stagnation leads to water binding. (气滞则水结 *Qi zhi ze shui jie.*)

Since qi moves water fluids in the body, qi stagnation may lead to water binding or damp accumulation.

Qi is able to transform dampness. (气能化湿 *Qi neng hua shi.*)

Because the qi moves and transforms water fluids in the body and dampness is nothing other than untransformed and nonmoving water fluids, qi is able to transform dampness.

Hundreds of diseases arise out of qi. (百病皆生于气 *Bai bing jie sheng yu qi.*)

Because qi is so important in the body, disorders of the qi is one of the main mechanisms of disease. In general, the qi can be vacuous or it can be depressed. When it is depressed, it can be stagnant, it may counterflow, and/or it may transform heat.

The ancestral qi is the stirring qi. (宗气者，动气也。 *Zong qi zhe, dong qi ye.*)

The ancestral or gathered qi is sometimes referred to as the chest qi. It is the combination of the heart and lung qi. It is the qi which stirs or propels the qi, blood, and body fluids throughout the body.

The ancestral qi is the place where the constructive [and] defensive unite. [It] exits from the lungs [and] accumulates in the sea of qi. (宗气者，营卫之所合也，出于肺，积于气海。 *Zong qi zhe, ying wei zhi suo he ye, chu yu fei, ji yu qi hai.*)

Because the lungs emit both the defensive and constructive qi, the ancestral qi is the place where these two unite. Further, the sea of qi is the chest or thorax.

The ancestral [or gathered] qi accumulates within the chest and exits from the throat. It passes through the heart vessels and moves inhalation [and] exhalation. (宗气积于胸中，出于喉咙，以贯心脉而行呼吸焉。 *Zong qi ji yu xiong zhong, chu yu hou long, yi guan xin mai er xing hu xi yan.*)

This statement explicitly says that the ancestral qi is located in the chest, exits from the throat, and empowers the heart and lungs.

The ancestral qi ascends [and] exits from the nose and makes for [the ability] to smell. (宗气上出于鼻而为臭。*Zong qi shang chu yu bi er wei xiu.*)

> This statement says that the ability of the nose to smell is dependent on the ancestral qi. Normally in Chinese medicine, we think that it is the lung qi which allows the nose to smell. However, since the lung qi is part of the ancestral qi, here it is said that the ancestral qi empowers the sense of smell.

[If] the ancestral qi does not descend, the blood within the vessels congeals, remains, and stops. (宗气不下，脉中之血凝而留止。*Zong qi bu xia, mai zhong zhi xue ning er liu zhi.*)

Qi transformation leads to the ability to exit [or discharge]. (气化则能出。*Qi hua ze neng chu.*)

> Urine, feces, and sweat normally can only exit from the body if the qi moves and transforms them. They cannot ordinarily exit the body by themselves.

The left side pertains to blood; the right side pertains to qi. (左属血，右属气 *Zuo shu xue, you shu qi.*)

> This is a yin-yang theory ascription. In clinic, we sometimes explain a right-sided headache as due to yang hyperactivity, while a left-sided headache may be due to blood vacuity.

The blood governs moistening. (血主濡之。*Xue zhu ru zhi.*)

> Nourishing and moistening are the two functions of the blood according to Chinese medicine.

Qi governs shining; blood governs moistening. (气主照之, 血主濡之。*Qi zhu zhao zhi，xue zhu ru zhi.*)

> Shining here refers to the warming and empowering function. Therefore, this statement clearly identifies the relative yin-yang duties of the qi and blood, shining being yang and moistening being yin.

The eyes obtain blood and are able to see. (目得血与能视 *Mu de xue yu neng shi.*)

The ears obtain blood and are able to hear. (耳得血与能听 *Er de xue yu neng ting.*)

The hair obtains blood and is able to gather. (毛得血与能聚 *Mao de xue yu neng ju.*)

The palms obtain blood and are able to grasp. (掌得血与能握 *Zhàng de xue yu neng wo.*)

The feet obtain blood and are able to step. (足得血与能步 *Zu de xue yu neng bu.*)

All these statements from the *Nei Jing (Inner Classic)* imply that any tissue or organ in the body can only perform its yang function empowered by its qi if that tissue or organ obtains adequate blood to nourish it.

The viscera obtain blood and are enabled by humors. (脏得血与能液 *Zang de xue yu neng ye.*)

The bowels obtain blood and are enabled by fluids. (腑得血与能津 *Fu de xue yu neng jin.*)

These two statements are a further clarification of the above. However, these two statements say that not only is nourishment by blood necessary for the organs to function correctly, they also must obtain sufficient fluids and humors to moisten them.

The blood [and] qi like warmth and are averse to cold. Cold leads to weeping and inability to flow, [while] warmth leads to dispersion and going. (血气者，喜温而恶寒，寒则泣不能流，温则消而去之。*Xue qi zhe, xi wen er e han, han ze qi bu neng liu, wen ze xiao er qu zhi.*)

Cold's nature is constricting and contracting, and the lumena of the channels and vessels must be relaxed and open for the qi and blood to flow freely. Therefore, the qi and blood like warmth and are averse to cold. If cold leads to lack of free flow and, therefore, pain, there is weeping or crying. Whereas warmth leads to the uninhibited movement and flow of the qi and blood.

When blood is exuberant, the hair is moist [*i.e.,* sleek and lustrous]. (血盛则发润 *Xue sheng ze fa run.*)

> Because the hair is the surplus of the blood, when the blood is exuberant or abundant, the hair is healthy. In clinical practice, dry, lifeless, falling, and/or prematurely grey hair are all common signs of blood vacuity.

The fountainhead of blood is located in the kidneys. (血之源头 在乎肾。 *Xue zhi yuan tou zai hu shen.*)

> Because it requires essence to engender blood and essence is stored in the kidneys, the kidneys may be said to be the fountain-head or spring of blood.

Blood is the essence of water [and] grain engendered [and] transformed by the spleen. (血者水谷之精也，生化于脾。 *Xue zhe shui gu zhi jing ye, sheng hua yu pi.*)

> Although the fountainhead of blood may be said to be the kidneys, the main viscus responsible for the engenderment and transform-ation of blood is the spleen. It is the spleen which engenders and transforms the blood from the finest essence of food and drink.

The color [of] the blood is the red color of fire. (血色，火赤之 色也. *Xue se, huo chi zhi se ye.*)

The color of the blood is only red [because] the heart fire transforms the blood. (血色独红者，血为心火之化。 *Xue se du hong zhe, xue wei xin huo zhi hua.*)

> These two statements explain why the blood is red in color. They state that the red color is due to the final transformation of the blood by heart fire or the heart's yang qi. Since the heart and the color red both correspond to the fire phase, the blood takes on the color red.

[If] the blood, the finest essence of water [and] grain, obtains the life-gate true fire's steaming [and] transformation, it engenders [and] grows the muscles [and] flesh, skin [and] hair. (夫血者，水谷之精微，得命门真火蒸化，以生长肌肉皮毛者也。 *Fu xue zhe, shui gu zhi jing wei, de ming men zhen huo zheng hua, yi sheng zhang ji rou pi mao zhe ye.*)

According to this statement, blood can only perform its function of engendering and growing the tissues of the body if it receives adequate warming and steaming from life-gate fire.

[If] the bones [and] marrow are hard [and] secure, the qi [and] blood [are] both plentiful. (骨髓坚固，气血皆从。*Gu sui jian gu, qi xue jie cong.*)

This statement seems to recognize that the bone marrow plays a part in the creation of blood.

[If] the blood is harmonious, [this] first leads to the grandchild network vessels [being] full [and] spilling over. Therefore [it] pours into the network vessels. [If] both are brim full, [it] pours into the channels [and] vessels. (血和则孙络先满溢，乃注于络脉，皆盈，乃注于经脉。*Xue he ze sun luo xian man yi, nai zhu yu luo mai, jie ying, nai zhu yu jing mai.*)

This statement posits an order for the blood to enter the channels and vessels. First it enters the smallest or grandchild network vessels (孙络, *sun luo*). Then it pours over into the regular network vessels, and finally it pours over into the channels and vessels. While this is an interesting idea, it is rarely used in clinical practice today.

The qi [and] blood of the elderly are debilitated, their flesh is dessicated, [and their] qi passageways are rough [or astringed, *i.e.*, not freely flowing]. (老者之气血衰，其肌肉枯，气道涩。*Lao zhe zhi qi xue shuai, qi ji rou ku, qi dao se.*)

Because of the decline of visceral function and the progressive consumption of essence due to age, qi and blood in the elderly are not engendered and transformed the way they once were. Therefore, their qi and blood tend to be insufficient to nourish and moisten their flesh and to keep their passageways smoothly and freely flowing.

[In] women, it is blood [which] makes [their] root [and] qi which makes for function. (女子以血为本，以气为用。*Nu zi yi xue wei ben, yi qi wei yong.*)

Because women menstruate, gestate, and lactate, they both use and lose blood in a way that men do not. Therefore, in women, the state of their blood is crucial to their well-being. Thus, in women, it is blood which makes their root.

Women's life has a surplus of qi [and] an insufficiency of blood.
(妇人之生，有余于气，不足于血。*Fu ren zhi sheng, you yu
yu qi, bu zu yu xue.*)

> This statement is a corollary of the above. Because of menstruation,
> gestation, and lactation, women often suffer from blood vacuity.
> This then creates a relative surplus of qi. However, this is only a
> relative surplus.

The blood within a woman's uterus is exchanged one time each
month, eliminating the old [and] engendering the new [or fresh
blood]. (女子包中之血, 每月一次，除旧生新。*Nu zi bao
zhong zhi xue, mei yue yi ci, chu jiu sheng xin.*)

> The blood that is discharged as the menstruate is not healthy, living
> blood. If conception has not taken place, it must be eliminated in
> order for the woman to engender fresh blood so she can try again.

[If] the sea of qi is full [and] exuberant, the heart is quiet [and]
the spirit is stable. (气海充盛，心安神定。*Qi hai chong sheng,
xin an shen ding.*)

> In this case, the sea of qi is the ancestral or gathered qi in the chest.
> If this chest qi is full and exuberant, then the heart spirit is
> constructed and fortified and, therefore, is quiet and stable.

Constructive & Defensive
(营卫, *ying wei*)

The constructive and defensive are two subtypes of latter heaven
qi which are both made from the finest essence of food and drink.

The constructive is located within the vessels; the defensive is
located outside the vessels. (营在脉中， 卫在脉外 *Ying zai mai
zhong, wei zai mai wai.*)

The floating qi which does not follow the channels is the
defensive qi. (其浮气之不循经者为卫气。*Qi fu qi zhi bu xun
jing zhe wei wei qi.*)

> This statement says that the defensive qi does not flow in the chan-
> nels. It also says that it "floats." This means that it floats to and trav-
> els in the exterior of the body.

The constructive exits from the middle burner. (营出中焦 *Ying chu zhong jiao.*)

> All sources agree that the constructive qi exits from the middle burner as the clear part of the finest essence of food and drink.

The defensive exits from the lower burner. (卫出下焦 *Wei chu xia jiao.*)

> According to some sources, the defensive qi exits from the lower burner. This is because it is also said that the defensive qi is created from the turbid part of the food and drink and the turbid is sent down to the lower burner.

The defensive exits from the middle burner. (卫出中焦, *Wei chu zhong jiao.*)

> Today, the standard theory is that the defensive qi exits from the middle burner along with the constructive qi. In this case, both are made from the clear part of the finest essence. However, the constructive is made from the clear of the clear and the defensive is made from the turbid of the clear. Thus we have the following two statements:

The clear becomes the constructive. (清者为营 *Qing zhe wei ying.*)

The turbid becomes the defensive. (浊者为卫 *Zhuo zhe wei wei.*)

The constructive [and] defensive are the essence [and] qi. (营卫者精气也 *Ying wei zhe jing qi ye.*)

> This statement means that the constructive and defensive qi are both made from essence provided by the kidneys and the latter heaven qi derived from food and drink.

The constructive is that which is the essence of water [and] grain; it harmonizes [and] regulates the five viscera [and] sprays [and] spatters the six bowels [like rain]. (营者水谷精气也，和调于五脏，洒阵于六腑 *Ying zhe shui gu jing qi ye, he tiao yu wu zang, sa zhen yu liu fu.*)

> This statement says that the constructive qi is made from the finest essence of food and drink and that it especially constructs and nourishes the five viscera and six bowels. The fact that it harmonizes and regulates the five viscera emphasizes the constructive qi

yang function on the yin viscera. The fact that it sprays and spatters the six bowels emphasizes its yin moistening function on the yang bowels.

The defensive qi moves within yang during the day [and it] moves within yin at night. (卫气者昼行于阳，夜行于阴 *Wei qi zhe zhou xing yu yang, ye xing yu yin.*)

The defensive qi travels in the defensive exterior during the day, warming the exterior and guarding against contraction of external evils. However, at night, the defensive qi retreats from the exterior of the body and enters the interior in order to warm the viscera and bowels. This is the Chinese medical explanation for many people feeling more easily chilled at night than in the day.

The constructive qi secretes [to form] the fluids [and] humors, [which] pour into the vessels, [which] transform the blood. (营气者，泌其津液，注之于脉，化以为血。*Ying qi zhe, mi qi jin ye, zhu zhi yu mai, hua yi wei xue.*)

According to this statement, the constructive qi engenders the fluids and humors which then enter the vessels and transform into the blood.

The constructive [and] defensive fill the place of the blood. (营卫者血之所充也。*Ying wei zhe xue zhi suo chong ye.*)

Based on the foregoing theory, the constructive and defensive fill the place of the blood, *i.e.,* the vessels. However, these last two statements are not commonly used in the contemporary practice of Chinese medicine.

What is called the constructive makes the blood, nothing else. Only the constructive qi transforms and makes the blood! (世谓营为血者，非也。营气化而为血耳！*Shi wei ying wei xue zhe, fei ye. Ying qi hua er wei xue er.*)

This statement says that the blood is made from the constructive qi, and certainly, the constructive and blood are closely related. For instance, in warm disease (温病, *wen bing*) theory, the last two of the four aspects or divisions warm hot evils progress through are the constructive and blood respectively.

Defensive qi guards the outside; the constructive [and] blood keep watch on the inside. (卫气外护，营血内守 *Wei qi wai hu, ying xue nei shou.*)

> The defensive qi flows mainly in the exterior (at least during the daytime), while the constructive qi and blood flow mainly in the interior. It is the defensive qi which guards against externally contracted evils, while it is the constructive qi and blood which maintain the health of the interior.

The constructive [and] blood enrich [and] nourish the entire body [as well as] the channels [and] network vessels. (营血滋养全身经络 *Ying xue zi yang quan shen jing luo.*)

> It is the constructive qi and blood which mainly flow through the channels and network vessels and which enrich and nourish all the tissues and organs of the body.

The defensive qi is hot qi. (卫气者，热气也。*Wei qi zhe, re qi ye.*)

> The defensive qi is hot in nature. Therefore, when the defensive qi becomes depressed in the exterior due to the presence of some externally contracted evils, the exterior becomes hot. In Chinese medicine, we then say that the patient effuses or emits heat (发热, *fa re*). This is often translated as having a fever.

The defensive qi is a hot qi which is able to warm the muscles [and] flesh [and] is able to transform water [and] grains. This is the function of the defensive qi. (卫气者，热气也，肌肉之所以能温，水谷之所以能化者，卫气之功用也。*Wei qi zhe, re qi ye, ji rou zhi suo yi neng wen, shui gu zhi suo yi neng hua zhe, wei qi zhi gong yong ye.*)

The defensive qi warms the divisions of the flesh, fills the skin, plumps the interstices, [and] commands [their] opening [and] uniting. (卫气者，所以温分肉，充皮肤，肥腠理，司开合者也。*Wei qi zhe, suo yi wen fen rou, chong pi fu, fei cou li, si kai he zhe ye.*)

> These two statements both say that the defensive qi is warm or hot and that its function is to warm the body. In the second statement, it also says that the defensive qi "plumps" the interstices. Plumping the interstices means to densely pack the interstices. This is the same as the defensive qi securing the exterior (固表, *gu biao*). By

closing the interstices, evils are shut firmly out. By opening the interstices, sweat is allowed to exit the body but evils are also more apt to enter.

The floating qi which does not follow the channels is the defensive qi. (其浮气之不循经者为卫气。 *Qi fu qi zhi bu xun jing zhe wei wei qi.*)

[If] the defensive qi is harmonious, the divisions of the flesh are untied [and] uninhibited, the skin is regulated [and] soft, [and] the interstices are resultingly dense. (卫气和，则分肉解利，皮肤调柔，腠理致密矣。 *Wei qi he, ze fen rou jie li, pi fu tiao rou, cou li zhi mi yi.*)

Fluids & Humors
(津液, *jin ye*)

Fluids and humors collectively refer to all the healthy or normal water fluids in the body. Comparatively fluids are thinner and clearer than humors which are thicker and more turbid. Thus fluids are yang to humors being more yin.

Humans are endowed with yin and yang, the two qi, in order to live, [and yin and yang] have clear [and they] have turbid. The clear of yang is the source qi, [while] the turbid of yang is fire. The clear of yin are the fluids [and] humors, [while] the turbid of yin are [things] like phlegm. (人禀阴阳二气以生，有清有浊。阳之清者为元气，阳之浊者为火；阴之清者为津液，阴之浊者即为痰。 *Ren bing yin yang er qi yi sheng, you qing you zhuo. Yang zhi qing zhe wei yuan qi, yang zhi zhuo zhe wei huo; yin zhi qing zhe wei jin ye, yin zhi zhuo zhe ji wei tan.*)
  According to this statement, fluids and humors are the clear part of the subdivision of yin into clear and turbid.

Fluids [and] humors come from the source of drink [and] food. (津液来源于饮食。 *Jin ye lai yuan yu yin shi.*)
  Fluids and humors are derived from the finest essence of food and drink.

Fluids [and] humors [exit] from the heart, pass through the lungs, fill [and] replete the skin [and] hair, [and] scatter through the hundreds of vessels. (津液于心，贯于肺，充实皮毛，散于百脉。 *Jin ye yu xin, guan yu fei, chong shi pi mao, san yu bai mai.*)
According to Li Dong-yuan, fluids and humors gather along with the blood in the heart. Then they pass through or are sent out from the lungs in order to fill the skin and hair, eventually scattering or dispersing through the hundreds of vessels.

[If] fluids [and] humors are harmonious [and] regulated, they change [and] transform becoming red to make the blood. (津液和调，变化而赤为血。 *Jin ye he tiao, bian hua er chi wei xue.*)
This statement likewise posits a connection between fluids and humors on the one hand and blood on the other. According to this statement, the blood is made from fluids and humors which have been turned red.

Fluids and humors are two types of different natured liquids. 津和液是两种不同性质的液质。 *Jin he ye shi liang zhong bu tong xing zhi de ye zhi.*)
This statement makes it clear that fluids and humors together form liquids, but they are of two different types.

The substance of fluids is mostly light [and] clear, while the humors... [are] thick, congealed, and bound. (津之质最轻清，而液。。。厚而凝结。 *Jin zhi zhi zui qing qing, er ye... hou er ning jie.*)
This statement defines the fluids as being very light and clear as compared to the humors which are thick, congealed, and bound.

The five visceras transform humors, the heart makes sweat, the lungs make snivel, the liver makes tears, the spleen makes drool, and the kidneys make spittle. [These] are the five humors. (五脏化液，心为汗，肺为涕，肝为泪，脾为涎，肾为唾。是为五液。 *Wu zang hua ye, xin wei han, fei wei ti, gan wei lei, pi wei xian, shen wei tuo. Shi wei wu ye.*)
According to this statement, it is the function of the five viscera which transform the five humors, and each humor is the product of a corresponding viscus according to five phase theory.

That which warms the muscles [and] flesh [and] fills the skin is the fluids; that which flows but does not move are the humors. (以温肌肉，充皮肤，为其津；其流而不行者，为液。 *Yi wen ji rou, chong pi fu, wei qi jin; qi liu er bu xing zhe, wei ye.*)

> According to this statement, the fluids flow through the skin, muscles, and flesh, while the humors flow but do not really move about the body. For instance, the humors make up the intra-articular and cerebrospinal fluids.

Sweat and urine both can be called fluids [and] humors. [If they are] replete, [they are] both water. (汗与小便，皆可谓之津液，其实皆水也。 *Han yu xiao bian, jie ke wei zhi jin ye, qi shi jie shui ye.*)

> According to this statement, sweat and urine are both species of fluids and humors, and fluids and humors when replete (in a good sense of being full and sufficienct) can both be called water.

Fluids [and] blood [share a] common source. (津血同源 *Jin xue tong yuan.*)

> This statement says that liquids in the body and blood both come from the same source, the food and drink taken in by the stomach and transformed by the spleen. Therefore, a vacuity of one may lead to a vacuity of the other. This is why, in clinical practice, we often add one or more blood supplements when we are trying to engender fluids and one or more fluid-engendering medicinals when we are trying to nourish the blood.

[If] water [is] diseased, blood [is] also diseased. (水病血亦病。 *Shui bing xue yi bing.*)

> This statement is the logical corollary of the previous statement. Because blood and liquids share a common source, disease of one can cause disease in the other.

For instance:

Deprived of blood, [there is] no sweating. Deprived of sweat, [there is] lack of blood. (夺血者无汗，夺汗者无血。 *Duo xue zhe wu han, duo han zhe wu xue.*)

[If] the movement of blood is not smoothly [or easily flowing], this causes dampness which results in stasis. (血行不畅，由湿致瘀。*Xue xing bu chang, you shi zhi yu.*)

Because blood and fluids move together, if the blood becomes static, fluids may collect and accumulate, transforming into dampness. However, this relationship is bi-directional. So dampness can also engender blood stasis.

Sweat [and] blood [share] a common source. (汗血同源。*Han xue tong yuan.*)

Because sweat is one of the five fluids, sweat and blood also share a common source.

The interstices effuse [and] discharge, the sweat exits [and] gathers together, [and this] is called fluids. (腠理发泄，汗出凑凑，是谓津。*Cou li fa xie, han chu cou cou, shi wei jin.*)

Yang added to yin is called sweat. (阳加于阴谓之汗。*Yang jia yu yin wei zhi han.*)

Sweat is referred to as yang added to yin because yang qi is necessary to effuse and emit the yin fluids which then appear as sweat. The sweat does not just fall out of the pores. It is transported from the pores by yang qi.

Essence & Spirit; Form & Spirit
(精神, *jing shen*; 形神, *xing shen*)

That which comes with life [or birth] is called the essence. (生之来，谓之精。*Sheng zhi lai, wei zhi jing.*)

Essence is what is inherited at conception from one's parents. In particular, this is the former heaven essence.

Essence is the root of the body. (夫精者，身之本也。*Fu jing zhe, shen zhi ben ye.*)

Essence is the most fundamental material substance making up the body. Therefore, essence is the root of the body.

Qi returns to [or gathers in] the essence. (气归精。*Qi gui jing.*)

There are two kinds of essence in the body, former heaven essence and latter heaven essence. As described above, former heaven essence is what we receive from our parents at the moment of conception. Latter heaven essence is manufactured from the surplus of qi and blood. Each day, we engender and transform qi and blood from the food and drink we take in and the air we breathe. This qi and blood is used to empower and grow or repair our body in all its daily activities. If, at the end of the day, we have made more qi and blood than we have used, when we go to sleep at night, this suplus is transformed into latter heaven essence. Some of this latter heaven essence is stored in each of the five viscera. However, the major portion is stored in the kidneys where it bolsters and supports former heaven essence. Therefore, the above statement is explaining how latter heaven qi gathers and is transformed into essence.

The qi [which is] not consumed returns [as] essence to the kidneys and makes essence. The essence [which is] not discharged returns to the liver and transforms the clear blood. (气不耗，归精于肾而为精；精不泄，归于肝而化清血。 *Qi bu hao, gui jing yu shen er wei jing; jing bu xie, gui yu gan er hua qing xue.*)

The qi [that is] not consumed gathers [as] essence in the kidneys and becomes [or makes] essence. The essence [that is] not discharged gathers as essence in the liver and transforms into essence blood. (气不耗，归精于肾而为精。精不泄，归精于肝而化精血。 *Qi bu hao, gui jing yu shen er wei jing. Jing bu xie, gui jing yu gan er hua jing xue.*)

These two statements specifically say that the unconsumed qi (and blood) is returned to the kidneys where it becomes (latter heaven) essence. They further say that essence is used in order to transform or make (liver) blood.

Essence transformed makes qi. (精化为气。 *Jing hua wei qi.*)

Essence is a form of stored qi and yin. Therefore, it can be transformed back into qi when needed. In addition, some essence is necessary to create the qi formed from the combination of the finest essence of food and drink and the great qi. Thus essence transformed makes qi.

Essence [and] qi engender each other. (精气相生。 *Jing qi xiang sheng.*)

> It takes essence to make qi, but it also takes qi to make latter heaven essence. Therefore, essence and qi engender each other.

Qi is life's sufficiency. Spirit is life's controller. (气者，生之足也。神者，生之制也。 *Qi zhe, sheng zhi zu ye. Shen zhe, sheng zhi zhi ye.*)

> According to this statement, qi is what creates life, but the spirit is what controls life.

A person's essence is the root of life. (夫精者，生之本也。 *Fu jing zhe, sheng zhi ben ye.*)

> One way of interpreting this saying is that, when a person's essence is completely consumed through the acts of living, there is the end of life. Another way to interpret it is that some essence is required in every act of engenderment and transformation in the body.

Essence [and] qi engender the spirit. (精气生神。 *Jing qi sheng shen.*)

> The spirit is nothing other than heart qi manifesting as the psyche and nourished and enriched by blood and essence. Therefore, essence and qi engender the spirit.

The spirit is the surplus of the qi. (神者，气之余也。 *Shen zhe, qi zhi yu ye.*)

Qi is to the spirit as the mother is to [her] child. Therefore, spirit congealing leads to qi gathering, [and] spirit scattering leads to qi dispersing. (神之于气，犹母之于子也。故神凝则气聚，神散则气消。 *Shen zhi yu qi, you mu zhi yu zi ye. Gu shen ning ze qi ju, shen san ze qi xiao.*)

> These two statements make it absolutely clear that the spirit is nothing other than an accumulation of qi.

Essence [and] qi nourish the spirit. (精气养神。 *Jing qi yang shen.*)

> Similarly, essence and blood nourish the heart qi or spirit.

The blood [and] qi [are] a human's spirit [which] cannot not be carefully nourished. (血气者，人之神，不可不谨养。*Xue qi zhe, ren zhi shen, bu ke bu jin yang.*)

> Given the above, one can say that, in fact, spirit is nothing other than qi nourished by blood. In addition, because of the spirit's importance to the proper functioning of the human being, it is extremely important that the spirit be adequately nourished.

The blood is the spirit qi. (血者，神气也。*Xue zhe, shen qi ye.*)

> Because blood constructs and nourishes the heart spirit and is indispensable to its existence and function, one can say that the blood is the spirit qi.

[When] the two essences assist each other, [this] is called spirit. (两精相傅谓之神。*Liang jing xiang fu wei zhi shen.*)

> The two essences are the former and latter heaven essences. Remember that latter heaven essence is formed from nothing other than abundant qi and blood. Therefore, the combination of latter heaven qi and blood and kidney essence are what form to create the heart qi or spirit.

Spirit is the essence [and] qi of water [and] grains. (神者，水谷之精气也。*Shen zhe, shui gu zhi jing qi ye.*)

> Because spirit is nothing other than qi accumulated in the heart and the heart qi comes from the finest essence of food and drink upborne by the spleen, one can say that spirit is the essence of water and grains.

Spirit is engendered from the qi, qi is engendered from the essence, essence transforms [into] qi, [and] qi transforms [into] spirit. Therefore, essence is the root of qi, qi is the ruler of spirit, [and] form [or the body] is the residence of the spirit. (神生于气，气生于精，精化气，气化神。故精者气之本，气者神之主，形者神之宅也。*Shen sheng yu qi, qi sheng yu jing, jing hua qi, qi hua shen. Gu jing zhe qi zhi ben, qi zhe shen zhi zhu, xing zhe shen zhi zhai ye.*)

> This passage further reiterates the relationship between essence, qi, and the spirit.

The five grains nourish, the five fruits assist, the five domestic animals boost, [and] the five vegetables fill. [When] qi [and] flavor [are] united and [one] administers [this, it] supplements [and] boosts the essence [and] qi. (五谷为养，五果为助，五畜为益，五采为充，气味合而服之，以补益精气。 *Wu gu wei yang, wu guo wei zhu, wu chu wei yi, wu cai wei chong, qi wei he er fu zhi, yi bu yi jing qi.*)

This passage explains again how food and drink supplement and boost the essence and qi.

The spirit is engendered by the essence [and] qi. (神由精气而生. *Shen you jing qi er sheng.*)

[If] the qi is harmonious and engenders, [and] fluids [and] humors are mutually produced, the spirit is therefore automatically engendered. (气和而生，津液相成，神乃自生。 *Qi he er sheng, jin ye xiang cheng, shen nai zi sheng.*)

These two statements again explain how the spirit is engendered out of qi and nourished and enriched by yin, blood, and fluids which, together, form essence.

[If one] obtains spirit, there is life; [if one] loses spirit, there is death. (得神则生，失神则死。 *De shen ze sheng, shi shen ze si.*)

When qi gathers there is life, and spirit is nothing other than the gathering of qi in the heart. Conversely, if one loses spirit, one has lost their qi and so has lost their life.

Superabundant spirit leads to smiling and laughing without stop; insufficient spirit leads to sorrow and pain damaging the heart. (神有余则笑不休，神不足则悲痛伤心 *Shen you yu ze xiao bu xiu, shen bu zu ze bei tong shang xin.*)

According to this statement, if one has abundant spirit, they will tend to be happy and smiling. However, if one's spirit is insufficient, one is apt to be plagued by sorrow and pain. In other words, those with abundant spirit suffer less, remembering that suffering is one's reaction to pain.

The form [and] spirit appear as one body. (形神一体观。 *Xing shen yi ti guan.*)

In certain instances, the concepts of form and spirit are juxtaposed as a yin-yang dichotomy. In this case, form refers to the body and spirit refers to the psyche. Therefore, the ancient Chinese were saying that there is actually no dualism between body and mind but together they form the living human being.

Form [and] spirit are united into one. (形神统一。*Xing shen tong yi.*)

The form [and] spirit [are] united [in] one. (形神合一。*Xing shen he yi.*)
These two statements are even more definite that form and spirit are actually one and that no dualism exists between them.

Form is engendered from no form. (有形生于无形。*You xing sheng yu wu xing.*)
Form is engendered by qi and qi is formless. Therefore, form is engendered from (that which has) no form.

Without form, there is nothing to engender spirit. Without spirit, there is nothing to quicken the form. (无形则神无以生，无神则形无以活。*Wu xing ze shen wu yi sheng, wu shen ze xing wu yi huo.*)

Form existing leads to spirit existing; form withering leads to lack of spirit. (形存则神存，形谢则神无。*Xing cun ze shen cun, xing xie ze shen wu.*)

Damage of form leads to dispersion of the spirit. (伤形则神为之消。*Shang xing ze shen wei zhi xiao.*)

The form [is] the tool which engenders the spirit. (形具而神生。*Xing ju er shen sheng.*)
All of these statements further clarify that the spirit is created by and is dependent on the functioning of the body. There is no ambiguity about this within Chinese medicine. The mind arises from the natural functioning of the body.

Essence is the root of the body. The form is the abode of life.

(精者，身之本也。形者，生之舍也。*Jing zhe, shen zhi ben ye. Xing zhe, sheng zhi she ye.*)

This statement essentially says that the essence is the root of the body, and the body is the house or abode of life.

The essence [and] qi of the five viscera [and] six bowels all ascends [and] pours into the eyes [which] are made by the essence. (五脏六腑之精气皆上注于目而为之精。*Wu zang liu fu zhi jing qi jie shang zhu yu mu er wei zhi jing.*)

As this statement posits, essence has a particularly close relationship to the eyes. In fact, the eyes are made from the essence of the five viscera and then are empowered by their qi.

The human spirit communicates with [and] responds to the great discipline of heaven [and] earth. (天地之大纪，人神之通应也。*Tian di zhi da ji, ren shen zhi tong ying ye.*)

This statement explains that, because the human spirit is nothing other than qi, it responds to the changes of heaven and earth or, in other words, the weather, the progression of day and night, the progression of seasons as well as changes in nutrition, etc.

[If] the mind is harmonious, then the essence spirit is focused [and] straight, the ethereal [and] corporeal souls are not scattered, regret [and] anger do not arise, [and] the five viscera do not receive evils. (志意和则精神专直，魂魄不散，悔怒不起，五脏不受邪矣。*Zhi yi he jing shen zhuan zhi, hun po bu san, hui nu bu qi, wu zang bu shou xie yi.*)

In Chinese medicine, the essence spirit as a compound term is the psyche and is basically synonymous with the spirit. Therefore, if the mind or psyche is focused and straight and is not disturbed by regret and anger, the five viscera function normally in their engenderment of righteous qi and, therefore, evils are not contracted.

[If] the blood vessels [are] harmonious [and] uninhibited, the essence spirit [has] an abode. (血脉和利，精神乃居。*Xue mai he li, jing shen nai ju.*)

This statement says that the essence spirit or psyche is healthy and well as long as the blood vessels are harmonious and their flow is uninhibited. In this case, one should remember that the heart is the abode of the spirit and the spirit is nourished by the blood. Further, the heart governs both the blood and the vessels.

[If] yin is level [or calm and] yang is secreted, the essence spirit [or psyche] is therefore in order [or at peace]. (阴平阳秘，精神乃治。*Yin ping yang bi, jing shen nai zhi.*)
In addition, if yin and yang are healthy and in harmony, then the psyche will also be healthy and at peace.

Thinking leads to the heart having a place [in which to be] preserved [and] the spirit having a place to return [to or gather]. The righteous qi is reserved and does not move. Therefore, the qi is bound. (思则心有所存，神有所归，正气留而不行，故气结矣。*Si ze xin you suo cun, shen you suo gui, zheng qi liu er bu xing, gu qi jie yi.*)
As we will see below in the chapter on disease causes, thinking makes the qi bind. Normally in Chinese medicine, binding of the qi is considered a bad thing. However, everything depends on degree. This statement says that a healthy amount of thinking helps to bind the spirit to the heart and thus the righteous qi is not scattered and dispersed. This statement shows that, in Chinese medicine, there is little that is either good or bad in and of itself. It all depends on degree.

Indifferent [and] not doing, the spirit qi [is] automatically full. (淡然无为，神气自满。*Dan ran wu wei, shen qi zi man.*)
This famous statement by Lao-zi says that, if one remains indifferent to the objects of perception and, therefore, doing nothing, the spirit qi is automatically full.

Unperturbed [and] indifferent [to loss and gain, believing in] nothingness, the true qi is obedient, the essence spirit abides internally, [and one is] always safe from disease. (恬淡虚无，真气从之，精神内守，病安从来。*Tian dan xu wu, zhen qi cong zhi, jing shen nei shou, bing an cong lai.*)
This statement advocating indifference to loss or gain and a belief in nothingness has clearly been influenced by Buddhism. Basically, it implies that the less the true qi or spirit stirs, the healthier it is and that, therefore, one will be safe from disease. The concept of nothingness (*sunyata* in Sanskrit) is a key concept in Buddhism, and

this concept had a definite influence on Chinese medicine during the Neo-Confucian period, the Song-Jin-Yuan dynasties.

Stillness nourishes the root of stirring, [while] stirring moves that [which is] still. (静者养动之根，动所以行其静。 *Jing zhe yang dong zhi gen, dong suo yi xing qi jing.*)

This statement says that stillness, being quiet and tranquil, nourishes the root of stirring, and it is qi which stirs within the human body. So stillness nourishes the engenderment and gathering of qi. *Vice versa*, it is the stirring of qi which moves all the substances in the body and animates the body which otherwise would be still.

Joy [and] happiness, the spirit dreads scattering and not being stored. (喜乐者，神惮散而不藏。 *Xi le zhe, shen dan san er bu cang.*)

According to this statement, joy is equated with happiness and happiness prevents the spirit from being scattered. This is because joy relaxes (缓, *huan*) the qi. When this word is applied to the movement of the qi, it means that it makes the qi move more slowly, however not slow enough to be pathological.

Joy leads to the qi [being] harmonious [and] the mind [being] broad; the constructive [and] defensive are freely flowing [and] uninhibited. (喜则气和志达，营卫通利。 *Xi ze qi he zhi da, ying wei tong li.*)

This statement further explains the effect of joy on the qi and, therefore, the spirit. Joy or happiness makes the qi flow freely and uninhibitedly.

[If] essence [and] qi are not scattered, spirit abides [and] is not divided. (精气不散，神守不分。 *Jing qi bu san, shen shou bu fen.*)

If the spirit is the gathering and accumulation of essence and qi in the heart, then it is important that this essence and qi are not scattered. Then the spirit can abide in the heart in a healthy and peaceful way.

Stillness leads to the spirit being treasured; agitation leads to [it] being dispersed [and] fleeing. (静则神藏，躁则消亡。 *Jing ze shen cang, zao ze xiao wang.*)

In Chinese medicine, agitation means fidgeting and physical rest-lessness and, therefore, stirring. Conversely, stillness is the lack of stirring or movement and qi is what makes stirring and movement. Thus the heart spirit or qi must move but it must not move too much.

Flavor returns to [or gathers in] the form, [while] form returns to the qi. (味归形，形归气。 *Wei gui xing, xing gui qi*.)
Flavor is the thick, turbid, or yin part of food which constructs and nourishes the physical body. However, the functioning of the body results in the engenderment of qi.

Qi returns to [or gathers in] the essence, [while] the essence returns to transformation. (气归精，精归化。 *Qi gui jing, jing gui hua*.)
As stated above, surplus qi is transformed into essence, but some essence is required in each transformation that takes place within the body.

Essence eats qi; form eats flavor. (精食气，形食味。 *Jing shi qi, xing shi wei*.)
Since surplus qi is transformed into essence, essence may be said to eat qi. Since flavor is transformed into form, form may be said to eat flavor.

Transformation engenders essence; qi engenders form. (化生精，气生形。 *Hua sheng jing, qi sheng xing*.)
The transformation of surplus qi and blood engenders essence, and it is the function of the qi that engenders the physical body.

Essence [and] blood [share] a common source. (精血同原, *jing xue tong yuan*.)

Essence [and] blood transform [into] each other. (精血互化。 *Jing xue hu hua*.)
Both of these two statements imply that essence helps make blood and blood helps make essence. Therefore, either one of these can transform into the other.

There are tai yin persons, shao yin persons, tai yang persons, shao yang persons, [and] persons [whose] yin [and] yang [are] level [and] harmonious. These five persons' constitutions are not the same. Their sinews [and] bones, qi [and] blood are each not equal. (有太阴之人，少阴之人，太阳之人，少阳之人，阴阳平和之人。凡五人者，其态不同，其筋骨气血各不等。*You tai yin zhi ren, shao yin zhi ren, tai yang zhi ren, shao yang zhi ren, yin yang ping he zhi ren. Fan wu ren zhe, qi tai bu tong, qi jin gu qi xue ge bu deng.*)

This statement has to do with why different people have different bodily constitutions. It divides bodies into five types: tai yin, shao yin, tai yang, shao yang, and those whose yin and yang are in balance. These different body types are different one from the other because they each have a different preponderance of yin and yang. Thus their sinews and bones, qi and blood are not the same.

Channels & Vessels
(经脉, *jing mai*)

The channels [and] vessels are the place for the movement of the blood [and] qi and the construction of yin [and] yang, the moistening of the sinews [and] bones, [and] the disinhibition of the joints. (经脉者，所以行血气而营阴阳，濡筋骨，利关节者也。*Jing mai zhe, suo yi xing xue qi er ying yin yang, ru jin gu, li guan jie zhe ye.*)

As this statement makes plain, the function of the channels and vessels are to circulate the qi and blood to the rest of the body and, in particular, moisten the sinews and bones and disinhibit the joints so that the body can exist and move in space.

The vessels have the extraordinary [and] common [or ordinary vessels]. The 12 channels are the common vessels. The extraordinary channels [are] the eight vessels. [They] are not restrained by the common [channels]. Therefore, [they are] called extraordinary channels. In terms of a human's qi and blood, [they] commonly move in the 12 channels [and] vessels. [If] these channels are all full [and] spilling over, [they] flow into the extraordinary channels. (脉有奇常，十二经者，常脉也；奇经

八脉，则不拘于常，故谓之奇经。盖以人之气血，常行于十
二经脉，其绪经满溢，则流入奇经焉。*Mai you qi chang, shi
er jing zhe, chang mai ye; qi jing ba mai, ze bu ju yu chang, gu
wei zhi qi jing. Gai yi ren zhi qi xue, chang xing yu shi er jing
mai, qi xu jing man yi, ze liu ru qi jing yan.*)

The two major divisions in the channel and network vessel system
in terms of therapy are the 12 regular channels (十二正经, *shi er
zheng jing*) and the eight extraordinary vessels (奇经八脉, *qi jing ba
mai*). As this passage explains, any surplus in the 12 regular channels
overflows into the eight extraordinary vessels. Therefore, the eight
extraordinary vessels act as reservoirs for the regular vessels.

The 12 vessels engender the 12 network vessels, [while] the 12
network vessels engender the 180 fastening network vessels. The
fastening network vessels engender the 180 winding network
vessels, [and] the winding network vessels engender the 34,000
grandchild network vessels. (十二经生十二络，十二络生一百
八十系，系络生一百八十缠络，缠络生三万四千孙络。
*Shi er jing sheng shi er luo, shi er luo sheng yi bai ba shi ji luo,
ji luo sheng yi bai ba shi chan luo, chan luo sheng san wan si
qian sun luo.*)

The 12 regular channels are paired with their 12 network vessels,
each channel having one network vessel. In addition, the governing
and conception vessels each have a network vessel, and then there
is the great network vessel of the spleen. So altogether there are 15
main network vessels. However, as this passage explains, these main
network vessels also branch into smaller network vessels and so on
until one comes to the smallest vessels in the body, the so-called
grandchild network vessels (孙络, *sun luo*).

The channels [and] network vessels govern the treatment of the
areas they pass through. (经络所过，主治所及。*Jing luo suo
guo, zhu zhi suo ji.*)

From the point of view of therapy, this statement is extremely
important. It says that diseases manifesting along the course of a
channel or network vessel can be treated by manipulating the flow
of qi and blood within that channel or vessel. It is this ability to treat
the channels and vessels that makes acupuncture effective. It is also
what allows for the stimulation of an acupoint to cure a pain or disease distant from it as long as the acupuncture point is on a channel
that does traverse the diseased area.

The vessel qi effuses at the points. (脉气发所之穴。 *Mai qi fa suo zhi xue.*)

This statement explains that the acupoints (穴, *xue*) are specific places on the channels where the qi is effused. The implication of this is that, by stimulating these places, one can affect the flow of qi and blood in the corresponding channels.

The channels govern the qi; the network vessels govern the blood. (经主气，络主血 *Jing zhu qi, luo zhu xue.*)

The implication of this statement is that one typically uses a fine needle (毫针, *hao zhen*) to stimulate the qi in the channels but uses a bleeding needle to stimulate the blood in the network vessels.

All superficial vessels [can] commonly be seen. (诸脉之浮而常见者。 *Zhu mai zhi fu er chang jian zhe.*)

Bleeding the network vessels is made easier by the fact that the network vessels which are typically bled can commonly be seen.

The 12 channels [and] network vessels internally home to the five viscera [and] externally network with the joints of the limbs. (十二经络者，内属于五脏，外络于肢节 *Shi er jing luo zhe, nei shu yu wu zang, wai luo yu zhi jie.*)

The interior (里, *li*) of the body is comprised of the five viscera and six bowels. The exterior (表, *biao*) of the body consists of the sinews and bones (筋骨, *jin gu*), muscles and flesh (肌肉, *ji rou*), and the skin and hair (皮毛, *pi mao*). As this statement makes clear, the channels and network vessels connect this interior with this exterior.

The internal pertains to the viscera [and] bowels. (内属于脏腑. *Nei shu yu zang fu.*)

This statement makes clear that the five viscera and six bowels comprise the interior.

The vessels are the mansion of the blood so that the qi has a root. (脉为血府，以气为本。 *Mai wei xue fu, yi qi wei ben.*)

Generally, when one talks of "vessels" in Chinese medicine, one is talking about the vessels which mainly carry the blood. Whereas, when talking about the passageways which mainly carry qi, one uses the word "channels."

[If] the blood vessels [are] blue-green [or cyanotic], inside there is static blood. (血管青者, 内有瘀血。 *Xue guan qing zhe, nei you yu xue.*)

   Blue-green, engorged superficial vessels are a sign of blood stasis.

The 12 channels [and] vessels move deeply between the divisions [of] the flesh. They are deep and cannot be seen. (经脉十二者，伏行分肉之间，深而不见。 *Jing mai shi er zhe, fu xing fen rou zhi jian, shen er bu jian.*)

   As this statement makes clear, the 12 regular channels are deep within the musculature and cannot be seen.

The passageways of the constructive qi treasure grains internally. (营气之道， 内谷为宝。 *Ying qi zhi dao, nei gu wei bao.*)

   The constructive qi travels within the channels. Therefore, the passageways of the constructive qi are the 12 regular channels. They can be said to treasure grains because the constructive qi is engendered from the finest essence of water and grains.

The essence [and] qi which move within the channels is the constructive qi. (其精气之行于经者为营气。 *Qi jing qi zhi xing yu jing zhe wei ying qi.*)

   This statement further makes it clear that it is the constructive qi made out of the finest essence of food and drink that primarily moves within the channels as opposed to the vessels.

The branches and horizontal [vessels] are the network vessels. (支而横者为络。 *Zhi er heng zhe wei luo.*)

   According to this statement, the network vessels tend to branch off and run horizontally between the regular vessels. Thus they connect the regular vessels, one to another, providing anastomoses, and also extending the circulation of qi and blood to the tiniest areas of the body.

The divergences exiting from the network vessels make the grandchild [network vessels]. Grandchild means to say they are small— the smaller and the more the better. (络之别出者为孙，孙者言其小也， 愈小愈多矣。 *Luo zhi bie chu zhe wei sun, sun zhe yan qi xiao ye, yu xiao yu duo yi.*)

This statement once again confirms that the main network vessels continue to branch and rebranch until one comes to the grandchild network vessels which are the smallest named vessels in the body.

The three yang are the *tai yang, yang ming,* [and] *shao yang.* (三阳者，太阳，阳明，少阳也。*San yang zhe, tai yang, yang ming, shao yang ye.*)

The 12 regular channels are divided into six yin and six yang channels. Then each of the six yang are divided into the hand yang channel and the foot yang channel. One hand and one foot yang channel make up a pair when talking about the six channels (六经, *liu jing*). Thus we can talk about the three yang channels and the three yin channels. Accordingly, the three yang channels are the *tai yang, yang ming,* and *shao yang.*

The three yin are the *tai yin, shao yin,* [and] *jue yin.* (三阴者，太阴，少阴，厥阴也。*San yin zhe, tai yin, shao yin, jue yin ye.*) This means that the three yin channels are the *tai yin, shao yin,* and *jue yin.*

The hand tai yin is the lung channel. (手太阴，肺经也。*Shou tai yin, fei jing ye.*)

The hand yang ming is the large intestine channel. (手阳明，大肠经也。*Shou yang ming, da chang jing ye.*)

The hand shao yin is the heart channel. (手少阴，心经也。*Shou shao yin, xin jing ye.*)

The hand tai yang is the small intestine channel. (手太阳，小肠经也。*Shou tai yang, xiao chang jing ye.*)

The hand jue yin is the pericardium channel. (手厥阴，心包络也。*Shou jue yin, xin bao luo ye.*)

The hand shao yang is the triple burner channel. (手少阳，三焦经也。*Shou shao yang, san jiao jing ye.*)

The foot tai yang is the bladder channel. (足太阳，膀胱经也。 *Zu tai yang, pang guang jing ye.*)

The foot shao yin is the kidney channel. (足少阴，肾经也。 *Zu shao yin, shen jing ye.*)

The foot shao yang is the gallbladder channel. (足少阳，胆经也。 *Zu shao yang, dan jing ye.*)

The foot jue yin is the liver channel. (足厥阴，肝经也。 *Zu jue yin, gan jing ye.*)

The foot yang ming is the stomach channel. (足阳明，胃经也。 *Zu yang ming, wei jing ye.*)

The foot tai yin is the spleen channel. (足太阴，脾经也。 *Zu tai yin, pi jing ye.*)

The yang ming governs the flesh; its vessel blood and qi are exuberant. (阳明主肉，其脉血气盛 *Yang ming zhu rou, qi mai xue qi sheng.*)
> The yang ming refers to the stomach and large intestine channels. According to this statement, these are the main channels which carry nutrients to the flesh. Consequently, the qi and blood within the yang ming channels is exuberant, meaning a lot.

The hand three yin leave the viscera [and] travel to the hands. (手之三阴，从脏走手。 *Shou zhi san yin, cong zang zou shou.*)
> The three hand yin are the heart, pericardium, and lung channels. Each of these channels arise from their corresponding viscera and travel down the ventral side of the arms to end at the tips of the fingers on the hands.

The hand three yang leave the hands [and] travel to the head. (手之三阳，从手走头。 *Shou zhi san yang, cong shou zou tou.*)
> The three hand yang are the large intestine, triple burner, and small intestine channels. These begin on the tips of the fingers on the hand and traverse the dorsal side of the arms to end at the head.

The foot three yang leave the head [and] travel to the feet. (足之
三阳，从头走足。 *Zu zhi san yang, cong tou zou zu.*)
 The three foot yang are the stomach, gallbladder, and bladder channels. These begin on the head, traverse the ventral side of the torso
 and the lateral side of the legs and dorsal side of the feet to end at
 the tips of the toes on the feet.

The foot three yin leave the feet [and] travel to the abdomen.
(足之三阴，从足走腹。 *Zu zhi san yin, cong zu zou fu.*)
 The three foot yin are the kidneys, liver, and spleen channels. These
 begin on the tips of the toes on the feet, traverse the medial side of
 the feet and legs and all three connect with their associated viscera
 in the abdomen.

The great network vessel of the stomach is also called vacuous
interior [虚里, *xu li*]. It passes through the diaphragm and networks with the lungs. It exits below the left breast [where] its
stirring responds [or can be felt beneath one's] clothes. It is the
vessel of the ancestral qi. (胃之大络，名曰虚里，贯膈络肺，
出于左乳下，其动应衣，脉宗气也。 *Wei zhi da luo, ming ri
xu li, guan ge luo fei, chu yu zuo ru xia, qi dong ying yi, mai
zong qi ye.*)
 The *xu li* refers to the apical pulse on the chest over the heart and
 indicates the state of the ancestral or chest qi.

The skin has [its] divisions [and] sections. (皮有分部。 *Pi you
fen bu.*)

All of the 12 channels [and] network vessels [have their] skin
zones. (凡十二经络脉者，皮之部也。 *Fan shi er jing luo mai
zhe, pi zhi bu ye.*)
 As these two statements say, the skin on the outer surface of the
 body is divided into zones which correspond to the 12 channels.
 These are referred to as the 12 skin or cutaneous zones.

[If one] desires to know the skin zones, mark the channels [and]
vessels. (欲知皮部，以经脉为纪。 *Yu zhi pi bu, yi jing mai wei
ji.*)

In order to map out the 12 cutaneous zones, all one has to do is trace the courses of the 12 regular channels on the skin. The zones are then the areas of the skin traversed by each channel and its surroundings.

That which are called the eight vessels do not fasten to the regular channels. Because yin [and] yang do not cooperate [in an] exterior [and] interior [way], [these] divergent pathways move strangely. Therefore, [they are] called extraordinary channels. (谓此八脉不系正经，阴阳无表里配合，别道奇行，故曰奇经也。 *Wei ci ba mai bu ji zheng jing, yin yang wu biao li pei he, bie dao qi xing, gu yue qi jing ye.*)

According to this statement, unlike the network vessels, the eight extraordinary vessels do not each attach to one of the 12 regular channels. Neither are they paired in an exterior-interior relationship as are the 12 regular channels. Because they are different from the regular channels they are called extraordinary, *i.e.,* not regular. However, this does not imply that they are clinically more powerful than the regular channels or that they possess some extraordinary abilities. They simply are unlike the regular channels in their courses and relationships.

The eight vessels home to the kidneys. (八脉属肾 *Ba mai shu shen.*)

According to this statement, all eight extraordinary vessels connect with or arise from the kidneys.

The conception vessel, *chong mai,* [and] the governing vessel [have] one origin but three paths. (然任脉，冲脉，督脉者，一源而三岐。 *Ran ren mai, chong mai, du mai zhe, yi yuan san qi.*) All three of these vessels originate in the uterus and emerge from the perineum.

The governing vessel governs the yang of the entire body. (督脉主一身之阳 *Du mai zhu yi shen zhi yang.*)

This statement means that the governing vessel governs all the yang channels of the body.

The conception vessel governs the yin of the entire body. (任脉
主一身之阴 *Ren mai zhu yi shen zhi yin.*)
The conception vessel then governs all the yin channels of the body.

The governing vessel passes through the upper back and homes
to the kidneys. (督脉贯背属肾 *Du mai guan bei shu shen.*)
This statement describes the anatomical course of the governing
vessel and that this vessel connects with the kidneys in a very
important way.

The conception vessel is the root of engenderment and nourishment in women. (任脉之妇人生养之本 *Ren mai zhi fu ren
sheng yang zhi ben.*)
Because women are heavily reliant on the state of their yin-blood
for both their health and function and the conception vessel governs all yin in the body, one can say that the conception vessel is
the root of engenderment and nourishment in women.

The conception [vessel] governs the uterus [and] fetus. (任主胞
胎。 *Ren zhu bao tai.*)
The conception vessel is one of the two main vessels which govern
menstruation and reproduction (the other being the *chong mai* or
penetrating vessel). Therefore, it is said that the conception vessel
governs the uterus and the fetus.

The penetrating and conception [vessels] are rooted in the blood
and home to the liver. (冲任本乎血而属肝 *Chong ren ben hu
xue er shu gan.*)
Because the penetrating and conception vessels are the two main
vessels that govern menstruation, it is said that they are rooted in
the blood. Because the liver and the blood chamber or uterus both
store blood, it is said that they home to the liver.

The penetrating [vessel] is the sea of blood. (冲为血海 *Chong
wei xue hai.*)
Again, this refers to the pivotal role of the penetrating vessel in the
regulation of menstruation.

The penetrating vessel homes to the liver [and] kidneys. (冲脉属
肝肾 *Chong mai shu gan shen.*)

Above we saw that all eight extraordinary vessels homed to the
kidneys. We also saw that the penetrating vessel in particular has a
close association with the blood. Since the liver stores the blood,
therefore the penetrating vessel is also said to home to the liver.

The penetrating [and] conception [vessels] arise within the uterus.
(冲任起于胞中 *Chong ren qi yu bao zhong.*)

Because both these vessels arise within the uterus and are associated with blood and yin respectively, they govern menstruation and
the conception and gestation of the fetus.

The penetrating [vessel] governs the sea of blood, [while] the
conception [vessel] governs all yin. (冲主血海，任主诸阴。
Chong zhu xue hai, ren zhu zhu yin.)

Here, we should understand this as the penetrating vessel governs
the blood, while the conception vessel governs the yin qi. Thus the
relationship of the conception vessel to the penetrating vessel in
terms of the regulation of menstruation and reproduction is that of
qi to blood.

The penetrating and conception [vessels] both start from within
the uterus, connect with the girdling vessel where [they are]
restrained, [and] flow freely to [or communicate with] the kidney
qi. (冲任俱起于胞中，受带脉所约，通于肾气。 *Chong ren ju
qi yu bao zhong, shou dai mai suo yue, tong yu shen qi.*)

This statement repeats two of the facts previously mentioned, that
these two vessels start from within the uterus and connect with the
kidneys. However, this statement also posits a connection with the
girdling vessel specifically for the purpose of restraining them. In
clinical practice, if the girdling vessel does not adequately restrain
the penetrating and conception vessels, there is abnormal vaginal
discharge flowing downward.

The penetrating vessel is the sea of the 12 channels. (冲脉者为
十二经之海 *Chong mai zhe wei shi er jing zhi hai.*)

The penetrating vessel is conceived of flowing through the core of
the body from the perineum to the crown of the head. Therefore,
it is similar to the axis of a globe. The channels are then arranged

longitudinally around the circumference of the body, somewhat like meridians on a globe. Because all the channels connect with the penetrating channel at the vertex, the penetrating vessel is the sea of the 12 regular channels.

[If] the two vessels of the penetrating [and] conception [become] vacuous [and suffer] detriment… [they will] not be able to control and restrain the menstrual blood. (冲任二脉虚损… 不能制约其经血。 *Chong ren er mai xu sun… nu neng zhi yue qi jing xue.*)

This statement makes their control over menstruation explicit. In particular, it also goes on to say that, if these two vessels are vacuous, the result with be meno- or metrorrhagia.

Debility [and] detriment of the penetrating [and] conception [vessels] leads to the menses not being free flowing. (冲任亏损则经事不通 *Chong ren kui sun ze jing shi bu tong.*)

This statement also ascribes menstrual disorders to vacuity of the penetrating and conception vessels.

[If] the penetrating [and] conception [vessels] are diseased, lactation will be insufficient. (冲任有病则乳液不足 *Chong ren you bing ze ru ye bu zu.*)

Lactation may be insufficient for either of two reasons. First there may be insufficient yin, blood, and fluids to transform the milk. Secondly, the free flow in the chest and breast region may be obstructed, thus preventing the discharge of milk. This statement does not specify either of these. However, because both vessels connect with the chest and breasts, if they are diseased, it may result in insufficient lactation.

If the penetrating vessel is diseased, there will be counterflow qi [and] internal tenseness [*i.e,.* cramping]. (冲脉为病逆气里急 *Chong mai wei bing ni qi li ji.*)

This statement specifically refers to abdominal cramping due to counterflow of the penetrating vessel. In actuality, this is a liver-spleen disharmony. It is ascribed to the penetrating vessel because such cramping is often treated by the meeting point of the penentrating vessel, *Gong Sun* (Sp 4), or by *Tai Chong* (Liv 3) whose name means the Supreme Penetrating (Vessel).

The qi and blood of all the 12 channel vessels [and] the 365 network vessels ascends to the face and travels to the cavities and orifices. Their yang qi ascends and travels to the eyes and makes their essence. (十二经脉，三百六十五络，其气血皆上于面而走空窍，其阳气上走于目而为之精。*Shi er jing mai, san bai liu shi wu luo, qi qi xue jie shang yu mian er zou kong qiao, qi yang qi shang zou yu mu er wei zhi jing.*)

> According to this statement, the qi and blood of all the channels and network vessels ultimately ascends to the head where it empowers and nourishes the clear orifices and especially the eyes.

All the vessels home to the eyes. [If] the eyes obtain blood, they are able to see. The essence qi of the five viscera and six bowels all ascend to pour into the eyes and make their essence. (诸脉者，皆属于目. 目得血则能见.五脏六腑之精气上注于目而为之精。*Zhu mai zhe, jie shu yu mu. Mu de xue ze neng jian.Wu zang liu fu zhi jing qi shang zhu yu mu er wei zhi jing.*)

> This statement reiterates the previous one, saying that all the vessels in the body connect with the eyes enabling the essence of the five viscera and six bowels to pour into them, enabling the eyes to see.

The head is the meeting of all yang. (头为者阳之会。*Tou wei zhe yang zhi hui.*)

> According to this statement, all the yang qi of the body ascends to the head. In the brain-ruling theory of consciousness, it is this accumulation of yang qi in the head or brain which empowers consciousness.

The channels [and] vessels are the place for enabling the determination of death [and] life, the management of hundreds [of] diseases, [and] the regulation of vacuity [and] repletion. [It is] not ok [for them] not [to be] freely flowing. (经脉者，所以能决死生，处百病，调虚实，不可不通。*Jing mai zhe, suo yi neng jue si sheng, chu bai bing, tiao xu shi, bu ke bu tong.*)

> According to this passage, the channels and vessels can be used for both diagnosis and treatment. They enable the determination of life and death. Hence they can be used for diagnosis. However, by regulating their vacuity and repletion, they can treat disease. Further,

it is especially not ok for their flow to be inhibited. They must be freely flowing in order for there to be health.

The essence of using needles lies in knowing [how to] regulate yin [and] yang. [If] yin [and] yang [are] regulated, the essence [and] qi are luminous, the form and qi are united, and the storage of spirit internally is promoted. (用针之要，在于知调阴与阳。调阴与阳，精气乃光，合形与气，使神内藏。*Yong zhen zhi yao, zai yu zhi tiao yin yu yang, tiao yin yu yang, jing qi nai guang, he xing yu qi, shi shen nei zang.*)

This passage states what acupuncture of the points and channels can accomplish. It can regulate yin and yang. By regulating yin and yang, the essence and qi are luminous and the form and qi are united. Hence the spirit is stored, with the assumption that there will be good health and long life. However, all this is based on the needles regulating yin and yang.

DISEASE CAUSES & MECHANISMS
(病因病机, *bing yin bing ji*)

Disease Causes
(病因, *bing yin*)

That which [produces] bitterness [or suffering] in a person is called disease. That which resulted in the disease is called [its] cause. (凡人之所苦，谓之病；所以致此病者，谓之因。*Fan ren zhi suo ku, wei zhi bing; suo yi zhi ci bing zhe, wei zhi yin.*)

In other words, there are diseases and their causes, and these are not one and the same. Disease causes are what initiates a disease. However, once initiated, one or more disease mechanisms are set in motion which then produce the signs and symptoms of the disease.

There are three causes: [that which is] called internal, [that which is] called external, [and that which is] called neither internal [nor] external. (其因有三：曰内，曰外，曰不内外。*Qi yin you san: yue nei, yue wai, yue bu nei wai.*)

The causes of any and all diseases can be divided into three types. Collectively, these are referred to as the three causes (三因, *san yin*). These three causes are internal causes (内因, *nei yin*), external causes (外因, *wai yin*), and neither internal nor external causes (不内不外因, *bu nei bu wai yin*). External causes are nothing other than the six (environmental) excesses (六淫, *liu yin*) plus pestilential qi (疠气, *li qi*), while the internal causes are nothing other than the seven affects (七情, *qi qing*). The neither internal nor external causes are an indeterminate list of such things as diet, lifestyle, sexual activity, poisoning, physical trauma, and iatrogenesis.

External Causes
(外因, *wai yin*)

Heaven [and] humanity correspond to each other. (天人相应 *Tian ren xiang ying*.)

> Because heaven and humanity correspond, humans may be affected by changes in the weather or other environmental factors associated with the six excesses.

The six qi result in disease. (六气致病。*Liu qi zhi bing*.)

> This statement explicitly says that the six qi or six excesses can cause disease. However, they usually only cause disease when they are excessive or untimely or if the person's defensive qi is insufficient. Therefore, the simple presence of the six qi do not always cause disease nor in everyone.

The six licentious [ones] are cold, summerheat, dryness, dampness, wind, and heat.[1] (夫六淫者，寒暑燥湿风热是也。*Fu liu yin zhe, han shu zao shi feng re shi ye*.)

> This statment lists the six excesses which may be contracted externally.

Heaven has six qi… [When] licentious, [these may] engender the six diseases. (天有六气。。。淫生六疾。*Tian you liu qi… Yin sheng liu ji*.)

> This statement makes it clear there is a distinction between the six qi of heaven and the licentiousness of these six qi which can then create disease.

---

[1] Wiseman *et al.* simply translate 六淫 (*liu yin*) as the "six excesses." However, 淫 (*yin*) literally means something morally loose or licentious. They are licentious because they cause disease when they are excessive or deficient for their season.

Wind
(风, *feng*)

Wind is the chief of the hundreds of diseases. (风为百病之长 *Feng wei bai bing zhi zhang*.)

Of the six excesses, wind is the most likely to cause disease. Therefore, wind is the chief of the hundreds of diseases.

Note: In Chinese medicine, wind means nothing other than an invisible, commonly airborne pathogen. It does not necessarily mean physical wind.

[If] there is damage, there must be wind. (有伤必有风。*You shang bi you feng*.)

This statement also underscores the tendency of wind to cause disease compared with the other five excesses.

[In] wind stroke, wind takes advantage of vacuity and causes disease. (中风，风乘虚而为病也。*Zhong feng, feng cheng xu er wei bing ye*.)

Wind stroke can mean either of two things. First it can mean any external contraction of wind evils resulting in disease. Second, it can refer specifically to a cerebrovascular accident (CVA) or stroke as a disease category. This statement can be read from either point of view. In the case of external contraction of wind evils, if the defensive qi is vacuous, wind evils may take advantage of this vacuity to enter and cause disease.

[If] the flesh is not hard [and] the interstices [are] sparse, there will be a tendency to disease [by] wind. (肉不坚，腠理疏，则善病风。*Rou bu jian, cou li shu, ze shan bing feng*.)

If the defensive qi is vacuous, then the interstices will not be densely packed nor will the flesh be hard. Thus wind evils easily enter the body to cause disease.

Prevalence of wind leads to stirring. (风盛则动 *Feng sheng ze dong*.)

Wind [and] fire [may] mutually fan [*i.e.*, exacerbate each other]. (风火相扇 *Feng huo xiang shan*.)

According to this statement, fire can give rise to wind but wind can also aggravate fire.

All wind with shaking [and] vertigo pertain to the liver. (诸风掉眩，皆属于肝 *Zhu feng diao xuan, jie shu yu gan.*)
This statement says that all wind causing shaking of the body and vertigo are due to internal engenderment of liver wind.

Wind prevailing leads to drawing [or pulling]. (风胜则引 *Feng sheng ze yin.*)

All fulminant rigidity pertains to wind. (诸暴强直，皆属于风 *Zhe bao qiang zhi, jie shu yu feng.*)
Fulminant rigidity means sudden, severe rigidity. This statement says such sudden, severe rigidity always involves wind. This wind may be either externally contracted or internally engendered.

Wind gives rise to parasites; dampness gives rise to parasites. (风生虫，湿生虫 *Feng sheng chong, shi sheng chong.*)
In this case, wind refers to an invisible pathogen. This is similar to the original Italian concept of malaria or "bad air" before scientists understood that malaria is transmitted by mosquitos. However, parasites are typically engendered in a damp internal terrain.

Cold
(寒, *han*)

Cold causes contracture [and] tension. (寒则收引 *Han ze shou yin.*)
This means that cold causes constriction and contraction of the channels and vessels and thus impedes the free and smooth flow of qi, blood, and fluids. It also means that cold often causes cramping and spasm.

Cold governs hypertonicity [and] shrinkage. (寒主拘缩。*Han zhu ju suo.*)
This means that cold is a main cause of all hypertonicity and shrinkage, contracture, or retracture in the body.

Cold leads to the skin [being] tense and the interstices blocked. (寒则皮肤急而腠里闭。 *Han ze pi fu ji er cou li bi.*)
  This statement is a corollary of the above. Because cold is contracting in nature, externally contracted cold evils cause the skin to contract or become tense and the interstices to become blocked.

Cold lodged by itself leads to blood congelation tears, [while] congelation leads to the vessels not being freely flowing. (寒独留则血凝泣， 凝则脉不通。 *Han du liu ze xue ning qi, ning ze mai bu tong.*)
  Cold leads to blood stasis and pain or tears. Blood congelation or stasis leads to non-free flow and inhibition of the vessels.

Diseases [with] watery humors that are clear, pure, and frigid pertain to cold. (诸病水液， 澄撤清冷， 皆属于寒 *Zhu bing shui ye, cheng che qing leng, jie shu yu han.*)
  Discharges that are clear and watery show a lack of heat and indicate the presence of cold. Typically, however, this is vacuity cold as opposed to externally contracted replete cold.

All cold with contraction [and] tautness pertains to the kidneys. (诸寒收引， 皆属于肾 *Zhu han shou yin, jie shu yu shen.*)
  This statement mostly refers to internally engendered cold due to kidney yang vacuity.

Cold evils depressed for a long time transform into heat. (寒邪郁久化热 *Han xie yu jiu hua re.*)
  Because the body's ruling or host qi (主气, *zhu qi*) is yang and, therefore, warm, if cold evils linger and endure in the body, they will eventually transform into heat evils. This is called similar transformation (同化, *tong hua*). According to this theory, any evil guest qi (客气, *ke qi*) will transform to become similar (*i.e.,* hot) to the host qi over time depending on the exuberance of the host qi.

Cold body [and] chilled drinks lead to damage of the lungs. (体寒饮冷则伤肺 *Ti han yin leng ze shang fei.*)
  According to this statement, being exposed to the cold can damage the lungs. In this case lung damage refers to an upper respiratory tract infection or common cold. According to this statement, drink-

ing chilled or iced drinks can also damage the lungs. However, this statement may be a cultural idiosyncrasy, since drinking chilled drinks is extremely common in developed countries and does not seemingly lead to catching a cold.

Cold prevailing leads to pain. (寒胜则痛 *Han sheng ze tong.*)
Because cold is constricting, it obstructs the free flow of the channels and vessels, and within Chinese medicine, the definition of pain is the lack of free flow. Therefore, cold prevailing leads to pain.

Extreme cold engenders heat. (寒极生热 *Han ji sheng re.*)
Extreme cold causes extreme constriction and, therefore, depression. In that case, depression transforms heat. Thus extreme cold engenders heat.

Cold damages the form, [while] heat damages the qi. (寒伤形，热伤气 *Han shang xing, re shang qi.*)
This statement says that cold primarily affects the physical body, such as in causing pain and cramping. Heat, on the other hand, damages the qi. This causes abnormalities in function and also causes qi vacuity.

Cold leads to qi contraction. (寒则气收 *Han ze qi shou.*)
Because of cold's constricting nature, it causes the qi to contract within the body, eventually leaving the extremities cold while attempting to maintain the warmth of the internal organs.

Cold exuberance leads to floating. (寒盛则浮 *Han sheng ze fu.*)
Exuberant cold in the exterior causes a floating pulse. This is because the defensive qi moves to the exterior to engage and try to eliminate the cold evils from the body. Hence the floating pulse evidences this struggle between righteous and evil in the defensive exterior.

Dampness
(湿, *shi*)

Water and dampness [are of] the same kind. (水与湿同类。*Shui yu shi tong lei.*)

Dampness is retained drink. (湿为留饮. *Shi wei liu yin.*)
These two statements say that dampness is nothing other than a pathological form of water. Internally engendered dampness is nothing other than unmoved and untransformed water fluids which collect and accumulate and transform into evil dampness. The second statement could also be translated as, "Dampness is lodged rheum."

Dampness is a yin evil whose nature is heavy, turbid, sticky, [and] slimy. (湿为阴邪，其性重浊粘腻。*Shi wei yin xie, qi xing zhong zhuo zhan ni.*)
This saying explains several things. First, it explains that dampness is heavy and, therefore, tends to seep downward in the body. Secondly, it explains that dampness is turbid. Therefore, even though dampness is untransformed water fluids, dampness cannot moisten the body tissues in a normal, healthy way. Third, because dampness is sticky, it is hard to eliminate. And fourth, because it is slimy, it impedes the free flow of qi.

Dampness by nature tends to descend. (湿性趋下。*Shi xing qu xia.*)
This statement corroborates the above in that it specifically says that dampness tends to descend.

[If] water collects, qi is obstructed. (水停气阻。*Shui ting qi zu.*)

Collection of water leads to obstruction of qi. (水停则气阻 *Shui ting ze qi zu.*)
The Chinese word translated in these statements as "collection" also means "to stop." So collected water is water which is not moving. Collection of water is a synonym for dampness. As this statement says, dampness obstructs the free flow of qi.

All tetany [and] rigidity of the neck pertain to dampness. (诸痉项强，皆属于湿 *Zhu jing xiang qiang, jie shu yu shi.*)
According to this statement, dampness is the main cause of tetany and stiff neck. However, while dampness may play a role in tetany and stiff neck, today these are not necessarily the main causes of these conditions.

All dampness [with] swelling [and] fullness pertains to the spleen.

(诸湿肿满，皆属于脾 *Zhu shi zhong man, jie shu yu pi.*)
This statement refers to both externally contracted and internally engendered dampness since it is the spleen qi which mainly must move and transform this species of evil. For instance, in clinical practice, we typically use medicinals which enter the spleen to treat all forms of dampness.

Dampness prevailing leads to pain. (湿胜则痛 *Shi sheng ze tong.*)
Because dampness obstructs the free flow of the qi and blood and pain is nothing other than the subjective sensation of a lack of free flow, dampness prevailing leads to pain.

Dampness prevailing leads to soft stool diarrhea; [if it is] serious, it leads to water block [and] bowel swelling. (湿胜则濡泄，甚则水闭腑肿 *Shi sheng ze ru xie, shen ze shui bi fu zhong.*)
Because dampness is heavy, it tends to seep downward from the middle burner to the lower burner where it commonly causes diarrhea. However, if dampness is so serious as to cause blockage to the movement of qi, it can cause water retention and swelling of the bowels.

Damp exuberance leads to yang [becoming] faint. (湿盛则阳微 *Shi sheng ze yang wei.*)
The spleen is the root of engenderment and transformation of the qi and yang is nothing other than a lot of qi in one place. Because the spleen is averse to dampness, exuberant dampness may damage the spleen, thus giving rise to a yang qi vacuity.

Damp depression transforms into heat; heat depression transforms into fire. (湿郁化热，热郁化火 *Shi yu hua re, re yu hua huo.*)
Because of the theory of similar transformation explained above, dampness may depress the movement of the qi. The qi then stagnates and transforms heat. Similarly, if heat becomes depressed, it may transform into fire, an even hotter form of heat.

[When] dampness [and] heat are mixed up, this causes dampness to transform into fire and fire to become toxins. (湿热昏淆，由湿化火，由火成毒 *Shi re hun xiao, you shi hua huo, you huo cheng du.*)

This statement explains how most toxins are engendered initially by damp heat. The dampness and heat struggle and the dampness causes the heat to become even hotter, transforming into fire. Then the fire boils and stews the dampness, transforming into toxins.

Fat people [have] lots of dampness. (肥人多湿。*Fei ren duo shi.*)
This statement says that fat people have more than normal amounts of dampness. This is internally engendered dampness. Below we will see that fat people do not only have excessive dampness but also excessive phlegm.

Summerheat
(暑, *shu*)

Summerheat is the ruling qi of the summer season. (暑为夏季主气。*Shu wei xia ji zhu qi.*)
This statement explicitly links the occurrence of summerheat to the season of summer.

Summerheat prevailing leads to earth [being] hot. (暑胜则地热。*Shu sheng ze di re.*)
If summerheat is exuberant, then the earth becomes hot, *i.e.,* the earth's weather becomes hot.

[In] this season, heaven [is] summerheat [and] the earth [is] hot. [Because] humans are in the center of these, contraction of these is called summerheat disease. (其时天暑地热，人在其中，感之皆称暑病。*Qi shi tian shu di re, ren zai qi zhong, gan zhi jie cheng shu bing.*)
During the summer, there is summerheat in the heavens and heat down on earth. Because people are located between these two, if they contract disease during this season, it is called summerheat disease.

Summerheat's nature is flaming [and] fire. (暑性炎火。*Shu xing yan huo.*)
Summerheat's nature is similar to fire in that it tends to flame and give rise to fire.

Summerheat's nature is upbearing [and] scattering. (暑性升散。 *Shu xing sheng san.*)

This means that summerheat tends to cause the righteous qi to ascend and disperse.

Summerheat months' heat damages the source qi. (暑月热伤元气。 *Shu yue re shang yuan qi.*)

This means that summerheat during the months of heat damages the source qi.

Summerheat leads to the skin [being] relaxed [or slack] and the interstices [being] open. (暑则皮肤缓而腠里开。 *Shu ze pi fu huan er cou li kai.*)

Summerheat is a form of external dampness specifically contracted during the summer months. According to this statement, its contraction leads to the skin being relaxed and the interstices open.

Summerheat mostly mixes with dampness. (暑多挟湿。 *Shu duo xie shi.*)

[If there is] summerheat, [there] must be simultaneous dampness. (暑必兼湿。 *Shu bi jian shi.*)

Summerheat and dampness [at their] source are two [different] qi. However, [they] easily are contracted simultaneously. (暑与湿原是二气，虽易兼感。 *Shu yu shi yuan shi er qi, sui yi jian gan.*)

It is very common for summerheat to mix with dampness. In that case, one talks of summerheat dampness. This means that the dampness of summerheat is more prominent than the heat of summerheat.

Dryness
(燥, *zao*)

Dryness is the ruling qi of the fall season. (燥为秋季主气。 *Zao wei qiu ji zhu qi.*)

This means that dryness is the ruling or background qi of the fall season, remembering that fall begins according to the Chinese calendar in the first week of August.

Dryness's nature is dry [and] rough. (燥性干涩。 *Zao xing gan se*.)

This means that dryness's nature is drying and, in terms of the human body, tissues which become dry also commonly become rough or chapped.

Dry qi damages the lungs. (燥气伤肺 *Zao qi shang fei*.)

Externally contracted dry evils typically attack the lungs and result in non-diffusion of the lung qi.

Dryness easily damages the lungs [and] reaches the liver. (燥易 伤肺及肝。 *Zao yi shang fei ji gan*.)

This statement begins by saying that dryness easily damages the lungs. However, it goes on to say such disease may eventually reach the liver, as when a dry heat condition in the lungs leads to a liver blood-kidney yin vacuity or when dry heat in the lungs negatively affects the movement of qi. Since the liver governs coursing and discharge, if such a lack of free flow reaches the liver, it may give rise to liver depression qi stagnation.

Dry exuberance leads to dry [symptoms]. (燥盛则干 *Zao sheng ze gan*.)

In other words, dryness leads to such dry symptoms as a dry mouth and parched throat, dry skin and hair, dry nose, dry eyes, dry vagina, etc.

Heat
(热, *re*)

Heat evils stir the blood. (热邪动血。 *Re xie dong xue*.)

Evil heat entering the blood aspect causes the blood to stir or move frenetically. This frenetic stirring may result in pathological bleeding.

Heat evils easily result in sores [and] welling abscesses. (热邪易 致疮痈。 *Re xie yi zhi chuang yong*.)

This means that heat is the main cause of all skin lesions and welling abscesses.

Where heat is excessive, blood becomes congealed [and] stagnant. (热之所过，血为之凝滞. *Re zhi suo guo, xue wei zhi ning zhi.*)

> Heat can cause blood stasis the same way that a stove's heat can turn milk into pudding. It stews the juices and thickens the blood until it congeals. Congealed blood is static blood.

All cramping, arched-back rigidity, and turbid water humors pertain to heat. (诸转反戾，水液浑浊，皆属于热 *Zhu zhuan fan li, shui ye hun zhuo, jie shu yu re.*)

> This statement can be read in two ways. The first is that cramping and arched-back rigidity with turbid fluid discharges pertain to heat. In this case, the statement refers to cholera. The second way of reading this statement is that all cramping and arched-back rigidity pertain to heat as do all turbid fluid discharges.

All sour retching [and] vomiting [and] fulminant downpour with lower body distress pertain to heat. (诸呕吐酸，暴注下迫，皆属于热 *Zhu ou tu suan, bao zhu xia po, jie shu yu re.*)

> This statement is describing acute vomiting and diarrhea as seen in acute gastroenteritis. It says that all such cases pertain to heat. However, in clinical practice, this kind of condition is usually due to damp heat, not just heat.

All abdominal distention and enlargement pertain to heat. (诸腹胀大，皆属于热 *Zhu fu zhang da, jie shu yu re.*)

All diseases [in which the abdomen gives forth] sounds and responds to tapping like a drum pertain to heat. (诸病有声，鼓之如鼓，皆属于热 *Zhu bing you sheng, gu zhi ru gu, jie shu yu re.*)

> Both these sayings state that all abdominal distention and enlargement pertain to heat. While heat accumulated in the stomach and intestines does cause abdominal distention and enlargement, heat is not the only cause of such distention. Therefore, this statement needs to be taken with a grain of salt.

Warm evils are contracted in the upper body. (温邪上收 *Wen xie shang shou.*)

Because heat is yang and yang inherently tends to move upward and outward, warm evils tend to be contracted first in the upper body.

Heat leads to the discharge of qi. (热则气泄 *Re ze qi xie.*)

Heat causes the qi to move more quickly and even frenetically. If the qi moves too quickly and scatters and disperses, it may result in the qi being discharged.

Heat exuberance leads to swelling. (热盛则肿 *Re sheng ze zhong.*)

Exuberant heat stews the body fluids and results in the accumulation of dampness. Dampness then leads to swelling.

Extreme heat engenders wind. (热极生风 *Re ji sheng feng.*)

Extreme heat may give rise to internal stirring of wind. If one has ever stood near a raging house fire, one can feel wind being sucked towards the fire. Likewise, forest fires typically give rise to their own wind.

Enduring heat damages yin. (久热伤阴 *Jiu re shang yin.*)

Chronic or enduring heat damages and consumes yin.

Heat harasses the heart spirit. (热扰心神。 *Re rao xin shen.*)

Heat damages the spirit brightness. (热伤神明 *Re shang shen ming.*)

Because heat naturally floats or flames upward and the heart is in the upper burner, heat may accumulate in the heart. In that case, the heat may damage the spirit by causing it to stir frenetically and/or by consuming it. Thus heat may damage the spirit brightness.

Heat damages the lung network vessels. (热伤肺络 *Re shang fei luo.*)

Similarly, because heat tends to float or flare upward and the lungs are the florid canopy, heat evils frequently accumulate in the lungs. If these heat evils are exuberant enough, they may damage the lung network vessels. Remembering that the network vessels contain blood, such damage causes hemoptysis or coughing up of blood.

Extreme heat engenders cold. (热极生寒 *Re ji sheng han.*)
Extreme heat eventually consumes the righteous qi, and the righteous qi is inherently warm. This then causes a yang qi vacuity with vacuity cold.

Fire
(火, *huo*)

Fire is extreme heat; warmth is gradual heat. (火为热之极; 温为热之渐。 *Huo wei re zhi ji; wen wei re zhi jian.*)
This statement explains the relationship between fire and heat and warmth and heat. Fire is simply an extreme form of heat, while warmth is a mild form of heat. These are issues of degrees, not of kind.

All six qi can transform [into] fire. (六气皆从火化。 *Liu qi jie cong huo hua.*)

Fire easily harasses the heart spirit. (火易扰心神。 *Huo yi rao xin shen.*)
Because fire is a form of heat, all heat in the body tends to float or flame upward, and because the heart is in the upper burner, fire easily accumulates in the heart where it harasses the heart spirit, causing the heart spirit to stir frenetically (动妄, *dong wang*). Eventually, such fire in the heart also leads to the consumption of the heart qi and, therefore, the wearing away or loss of heart spirit.

All clenching, shuddering, [and] chattering [of the jaws] with seeming loss of the spirit's vigil pertain to fire. (诸禁鼓栗, 如丧神守，皆属于火 *Zhu jin gu li, ru sang shen shou, jie shu yu huo.*)
This statement is describing febrile convulsions and deranged speech or delirium. According to this statement, fire evils accumulated in the pericardium are harassing the heart spirit and causing major chaos in the flow of qi and blood.

All agitation and mania pertain to fire. (诸躁狂越，皆属于火 *Zhu zao kuang yue, jie shu yu huo.*)

This means that all agitation and mania are due to heat or fire evils harassing the heart spirit. This is a reliable saying in clinical practice.

Fire easily damages fluids [and] consumes the qi. (火易伤津耗气。 *Huo yi shang jin hao qi.*)

Because fire is an extreme form of yang and fluids are yin, fire easily damages and consumes fluids, thus leading to yin vacuity and fluid dryness signs and symptoms. Fire also consumes and damages qi, leading to qi vacuity.

All diseases [with] superficial swelling, aching [and] soreness, [and] fright [and] astonishment pertain to fire. (诸病浮肿，疼酸惊骇，皆属于火 *Zhu bing fu zhong, teng suan jing hai, jie shu yu huo.*)

While superficial edema with aching and soreness may be due to other causes, the fright and astonishment indicate that fire evils are harassing the heart spirit.

All heat with visual distortion [and] spasm pertain to fire. (诸热瞀瘛，皆属于火 *Zhu re mao chi, jie shu yu huo.*)

In this statement, heat may be read as fever. Therefore, fever with visual distortions and spasms are due to fire harassing above.

All counterflow upsurging pertains to fire. (诸逆冲上，皆属于火 *Zhu ni chong shang, jie shu yu huo.*)

The implication of this statement is that fire surging upward to the heart is due to life-gate/ministerial fire counterflowing upward. Li Dong-yuan referred to this as yin fire (阴火, *yin huo*).

Fire and the source qi cannot both exist; [if] one prevails, one [*i.e.*, the other] loses. (火与元气不两立，一胜则一负 *Huo yu yuan qi bu liang li, yi sheng ze yi fu.*)

In this statement made by Li Dong-yuan, fire refers to yin fire and source qi refers to the central qi which is the latter heaven source. What Li is saying is that, if yin fire counterflows upward from the lower into the middle burner, it damages the spleen qi. However, if the spleen qi is fortified and exuberant, this yin fire cannot stir upward and leave its lower source (下原, *xia yuan*).

Fire depression leads to reversal. (火郁则厥 *Huo yu ze jue.*)
Fire depression refers to qi depression transforming not just into heat but into fire. In this case, the fire may be depressed within the interior of the body leaving the extremities and outer part of the body cold and chilled. Such exterior cold but interior warmth is sometimes referred to as reversal. In that case, the pulse will tend to be rapid and the tongue will tend to be red with yellow fur.

Fire depression [causes] the network vessels of the eyes to be parched. (火郁者络目燥 *Huo yu zhe luo mu zao.*)
Fire depression typically occurs in the liver due to liver depression qi stagnation, and the eyes are the orifices of the liver, connected to the liver by an internal pathway. If the heat of this fire depression in the liver follows this channel upwards to the eyes, the heat may damage the network vessels in the eyes. The network vessels carry blood, and blood and fluids share a common source and move together. Therefore, this heat may damage the blood and fluids which moisten the eyes, resulting in dry eyes.

Fire scurrying leads to hypertonicity. (火窜则挛 *Huo cuan ze luan.*)
Fire scurrying about the body may damage blood and yin fluids which then fail to nourish and moisten the sinews. The sinews then become dry and contract, leading to hypertonicity.

Exuberant fire leads to withering of fluids; fire depression engenders phlegm. (火盛则津枯，火郁生痰 *Huo sheng ze jin ku, huo yu sheng tan.*)
The first part of this statement means that exuberant fire damages yin fluids and leads to fluid dryness and dry signs and symptoms. In the second part, fire depression implies that there is a combination of fire and stagnant or depressed qi. In that case, the fire stews the juices and congeals them into phlegm, while the depressed qi fails to move water fluids which collect and transform, also congealing into phlegm. Therefore, fire depression is a two-fold mechanism for engendering phlegm.

Vigorous fire eats qi. (壮火食气 *Zhuang huo shi qi.*)
This means that exuberant or vigorous fire damages the qi leading it to become vacuous.

Fire is the root of rashes. Rashes are fire's sprout. (火为疹之根，疹为火之苗。 *Huo wei zhen zhi gen, zhen wei huo zhi miao.*)

> If pathological heat or fire enter the blood aspect, they may cause blood heat. In that case, the blood moves frenetically and may move to the exterior of the body where it causes red rashes. In that case, rashes are fire's sprout.

The origin [of] welling [and] flat abscesses is the engenderment [of] fire toxins [which] obstruct [and] separate the channels [and] network vessels [and cause] congelation of the qi [and] blood. (痈疽原是火毒生，经络阻隔气血凝。 *Yong ju yuan shi huo du sheng, jing luo zu ge qi xue ning.*)

> If fire boils and brews, stewing the juices, it may give rise to the engenderment of toxins. Further, if those fire toxins obstruct the free flow of the channels and network vessels, congealing the blood and stagnating the qi, they may give rise to welling or flat abscesses.

Skinny people [have] lots of fire. (瘦人火多也。 *Shou ren huo duo ye.*)

> This means that people who are skinny or thin tend to have lots of heat, not necessarily fire.

Internal Causes
(内因, *nei yin*)

The affects [and] mind quicken [and] stir. (情志活动。 *Qing zhi huo dong.*)

> This means that the movement of the qi associated with the affects and the workings of the mind can cause disruption to the functions of the viscera internally.

Anger leads the qi to ascend. (怒则气上 *Nu ze qi shang.*)

> According to this statement, anger causes the qi to move upward in the body.

Fulminant anger damages the liver. (暴怒伤肝 *Bao nu shang gan.*)

> Because anger is the affect or orientation of the liver, great or fulminant anger damages the liver. According to Qin Bo-wei, fulminant anger, *i.e.,* anger that has been let loose, is a species of

over-coursing and over-discharge. Because anything that is either too much or too little can cause disease, over-coursing and over-discharge damage the liver. The end result of this damage is that the liver becomes depressed and the qi becomes stagnant.

Fulminant anger damages yin. (暴怒伤阴 *Bao nu shang yin.*)

This statement can be read in either of two ways. First, fulminant anger may damage the liver which is a yin viscus. Secondly, fulminant anger may give rise to heat or fire which damages and consumes yin.

Great anger leads to the form [and] color being cut off [and] blood meandering above. (大努则形色绝，血宛于上。*Da nu ze xing se jue, xue wan yu shang.*)

This statement is an explanation of why the face gets red when one is extremely angry. According to this statement, great anger causes the blood to move upward to the face.

Having angry qi damages the liver. [Thus] the liver horizontally breaches [and] causes the blood not to be stored. (有怒气伤肝，肝气横决，血因不藏。*You nu qi shang gan, gan qi heng jue, xue yin bu cang.*)

According to this statement, anger results in liver depression. The liver then counterflows horizontally to assail the spleen. The spleen qi becomes vacuous and loses its control over the containment of the blood. Thus there is bleeding. This is what is meant here by the blood not being stored.

Joy leads to the qi becoming relaxed. (喜则气缓 *Xi ze qi huan.*)

In this case, joy means happiness, and happiness results in relaxation. Mostly this is a good thing, and, as such, happiness or joy is the antidote to all the other six affects. However, in extreme, happiness may cause too much relaxation which then negatively affects the flow of the qi, blood, and fluids.

Fulminant joy damages yang. (暴喜伤阳 *Bao xi shang yang.*)

In this case, fulminant joy means excessive mental-emotional excitation. This causes the qi and, therefore, yang to move frenetically, and such frenetic movement may result in the draining and discharge of the yang qi. Thus fulminant joy may damage yang.

Sorrow leads to the qi dispersing. (悲则气消。 *Bei ze qi xiao.*)
According to five phase theory, sorrow is the affect of the lungs, and the lung qi should accumulate in the chest. However, too much sorrow disperses the qi.

Fright leads to chaotic qi. (惊则气乱 *Jing ze qi luan.*)
Fright means a sudden startle or fright, as when one jumps because of a banging door or someone sneaking up behind one. Therefore, it is not hard to understand how fright causes the qi to become chaotic. When we are startled, all our qi moves outward suddenly and fails to gather or collect.

Fright makes the heart diseased. (惊为心病。 *Jing wei xin bing.*)
In particular, this statement says that fright makes the heart diseased. However, this means constant, repetitive fright as in war. It does not mean that a single everyday fright damages the heart.

Thought leads to binding of the qi. (思则气结 *Si ze qi jie.*)
While a certain amount of thought leads to a good gathering or binding of the qi within the body, excessive thinking leads to pathological binding of the qi. Notice also that this binding has nothing to do with good or bad thoughts. It is the process of thinking itself that is being talked about here. Further, because thought is not an emotion, this is why we cannot translate the Chinese word 情 (*qing*) as emotion when talking about the seven affects.

Fear leads the qi downward. (恐则气下 *Kong ze qi xia.*)
In Chinese medicine, fear is fear of something which has not yet happened or is not yet in one's immediate presence. According to Chinese medicine, fear causes the qi to move downward in the body. In English, we talk about fear causing a "sinking feeling." Certainly, we all know that excessive fear can cause uncontrolled defecation and/or urination, both of which are manifestations of qi moving downward.

Fear damages the kidneys. (恐伤肾 *Kong shang shen.*)
Because fear corresponds to the kidneys according to five phase theory, excessive or great fear can eventually damage the kidneys.

Unresolved fear [and] dread lead to damage of the essence. (恐惧而不解则伤精。*Kong ju er bu jie ze shang jing.*)

> If fear and dread go on for a long time, they lead to damage of the essence. To understand this statement, one should think of post-traumatic stress disorder (PTSD) due to unremitting great fear and recurrent fright. In this case, we can say that the unresolved fear and dread have damaged the essence which then does not nourish and keep the spirit qi healthy.

Fear is yang [and] goes from outside to inside; fright is yin [and] goes from inside to outside. Fear is from something unknown; fright is from something known. (恐者为阳，从外入也；惊者为阴，从内出也。恐者，为自不知故也；惊者，自知也。*Kong zhe wei yang, cong wai ru ye; jing zhe wei yin, ru nei chu ye. Kong zhe, wei zi bu zhi gu ye; jing zhe, zi zhi ye.*)

> This statement explains the differences between fear and fright in Chinese medicine. Fear causes the qi to sink, *i.e.*, travel from outside to inside, while fright causes the qi to move from inside to outside. Fear is of something unknown, while fright is due to actual present stimuli.

If joy and anger are not restrained, yin qi will counterflow upward; if there is counterflow above, there will be vacuity below. (喜怒不节则阴气上逆，上逆则下虚 *Xi nub u jie ze yin qi shang ni, shang ni ze xia xu.*)

> Joy as excitement and anger can both cause the qi to ascend. If this causes the kidney or yin qi to counterflow upward, there is repletion above but vacuity below.

Joy and anger damage the qi; cold and summerheat damage the form. (喜怒伤气，寒暑伤形 *Xi nu shang qi, han shu shang xing.*)

> According to this statement, excitement and anger primarily damage the qi or function, while cold and summerheat can damage the physical body.

Internal damage by anxiety [and] anger leads the qi to counterflow upward. (内伤于忧努，则气上逆。*Nei shang yu you nu, ze qi shang ni.*)

> According to this statement, anxiety can also cause the qi to counterflow upward, not just anger and/or excitement.

The five orientations [*i.e.,* emotions] transform into fire. (五志化火 *Wu zhi hua huo.*)

All the five orientations (*i.e.*, emotions) when extreme are able to generate fire. (五志过极皆能生火 *Wu zhi guo ji jie neng sheng huo.*)

Damage of the affects [*i.e.,* emotions] all lead to [diseases] pertaining to fire and heat. (情之所伤，则皆属火热 *Qing zhi suo shang, ze jie shu huo re.*)

> These three statements all say that extremes of any of the five affects may result in the engenderment and transformation of heat or fire.

[If] the mind's desires are not satisfied, the liver qi [becomes] depressed [and] bound. (情志不遂，肝气郁结。 *Qing zhi bu sui, gan qi yu jie.*)

> All desires are the subjective experience of the movement of the qi towards or away from something. Therefore, if desires are not fulfilled, the qi is not freely flowing. In that case, the liver's governance of coursing and discharge is damaged resulting in liver depression qi stagnation.

Speaking [and] laughing without limit, thinking [and] pondering supreme [and] deep, all [cause] detriment to the years of one's long life. (语笑无度，思虑太深，皆损年寿。 *Yu xiao wu du, si lu tai shen, jie sun nian shou.*)

> According to this statement by Sun Si-miao, too much speaking, laughing, thinking, and worrying can all shorten one's lifespan.

[If one] understands sufficiency, one is constantly happy. (知足者常乐。 *Zhi zu zhe chang le.*)

> According to this statement, if one understands the concept of sufficiency or enough, then one is constantly happy.

Neither Internal Nor External Causes
(不内不外因, *bu nei bu wai yin*)

Diet
(饮食, *yin shi*, literally drink [and] food)

The root of a quiet body must be supplied by food. (安身之本, 必资于食。*An shen zhi ben, bi zi yu shi.*)
According to this saying by Sun Si-maio, the root of good health depends on proper diet.

[When] eating, it is not ok to become over full. (食不可过饱。 *Shi bu ke guo bao.*)
One should not eat until stuffed.

Great stuffing blocks the blood vessels. (大饱血脉闭。*Da bao xue mai bi.*)
According to this statement, overeating leads to blockage of the blood vessels.

Hunger leads to damage of the qi. (饥则伤气。*Ji ze shang qi.*)
Here we are not talking about normal hunger. Here we are talking about being famished or starved. According to this statement, such extreme hunger leads to damage of the qi.

Lack of discipline in drinking [and] eating leads to stomach disease. (饮食不节则胃病 *Yin shi bu jie ze wei bing.*)
Because the stomach takes in the food and drink, it is the first organ to be affected by faulty, unregulated diet. In particular, overeating causes food stagnation (食滞, *shi zhi*) in the stomach.

[If] drinking [and] eating lose their discipline, cold [and] warmth will not be proper [and] the spleen [and] stomach will therefore be damaged. (饮食失节, 寒温不识。脾胃乃伤 *Yin shi shi jie, han wen bu shi, pi wei nai shang.*)
If one eats too many hot or cold natured foods, then cold and warmth will not be proper. In that case, overeating hot foods will cause heat to accumulate in the stomach, while overeating cold foods will damage the spleen and cause it to become vacuous.

[If] grains do not enter, [in] half a day, the qi declines [and in] one day, the qi is scanty. (谷不入，半日则气衰，一日则气少矣。 *Gu bu ru, ban ri ze qi shuai, yi ri ze qi shao yi.*)

According to this statement, one's qi will already have declined or gotten less if one does not eat for half a day. If one does not eat for a whole day, then one's qi is actually scanty or appreciably less than normal.

[If] drinking [and] eating are doubled, the intestines [and] stomach are damaged. (饮食自倍，肠胃乃伤。 *Yin shi zi bei, chang wei nai shang.*)

This means that overeating damages the stomach and intestines.

Drinking [and] eating, taxation [and] fatigue lead to damage of the spleen. (饮食，劳倦，则伤脾。 *Yin shi, lao juan, ze shang pi.*)

Either faulty diet or overtaxation and fatigue may damage the spleen causing its qi to become vacuous and weak.

Hot food damages the bones; chilled food damages the lungs. (热食伤骨，冷食伤肺。 *Re shi shang gu, leng shi shang fei.*)

According to Sun Si-miao, overeating hot foods damages the bones, while overeating chilled foods damages the lungs.

Enduring drinking of alcohol rottens [and causes] festering [in] the intestines [and] stomach. (久饮酒者，腐烂肠胃. *Jiu yin jiu zhe, fu lan chang wei.*)

According to this statement, long-time over-drinking of alcohol causes rottening and festering, *i.e.*, ulceration, in the stomach and intestines.

Lifestyle
(动静, *dong jing*, literally stirring [and] stillness)

Movement of the body gladdens the spirit. (动形怡神。 *Dong xing yi shen.*)

This statement says that a moderate amount of physical exercise is good for the spirit. In this case, the word 怡 (*yi*) means to both make happy and make relaxed or at ease.

[If] the form [or body does] not stir, the essence [will] not flow. [If] the essence [does] not flow, the qi [becomes] depressed. (形不动则精不流，精不流则气郁。*Xing bu dong ze jing bu liu, jing bu liu ze qi yu.*)

This statement says that lack of stirring or physical exercise results in the qi becoming depressed or stagnant.

Taxation leads to consumption of qi. (劳则耗气 *Lao ze hao qi.*)

Taxation means overwork, and overwork leads to consumption of the qi.

Physical overtaxation [and] labor lead to spleen disease. (形体劳役则脾病 *Xing ti lao yi ze pi bing.*)

Because the spleen is the latter heaven root of the engenderment and transformation of the qi and the qi is consumed if the body overworks and becomes too fatigued, overtaxation damages the spleen and causes it to become vacuous.

Taxation [and] vexation damage yang, [and] yang vacuity leads to gathering of drinks [*i.e.,* fluids]. (劳烦伤阳，阳虚则饮聚 *Lao fan shang yang, yang xu ze yin ju.*)

According to this statement, both taxation and vexation damage the yang qi, leading to yang qi vacuity. However, it is the yang qi which moves and transforms water fluids in the body. Therefore, if yang qi becomes vacuous, water fluids will not be moved and transformed. Instead they will collect and transform into dampness.

A lot of speaking leads to lack of qi. (多语则气乏。*Duo yu ze qi fa.*)

A lot of speaking damages the qi. (多言伤气 *Duo yan shang qi.*)

Speech is empowered by the exhalation of qi from the lungs. Therefore, excessive speaking damages the qi. This includes singing and chanting as well. In fact, excessive speech is so deleterious to the health that Li Dong-yuan said that, although he could not control all of his life's activities, he intended to preserve his health just by not speaking so much.

Prolonged looking damages the blood. (久视伤血 *Jiu shi shang xue.*)

Prolonged looking mostly means prolonged reading. Because it is the blood which enables the eyes to see, prolonged looking consumes or damages the blood. Conversely, once the blood has been damaged, the eyes no longer see so well and there is decreased vision. This is Chinese medicine's explanation why prolonged reading and meticulous eye work can result in decreased eyesight.

Prolonged lying damages the qi. (久卧伤气 *Jiu wo shang qi.*)

Because of prolonged lying the qi does not circulate. Instead, it becomes depressed, and qi depression may lead to spleen vacuity and its consequent lack of engenderment of the qi. Therefore, prolonged lying damages the qi by causing qi stagnation and/or qi vacuity.

Prolonged standing damages the bones. (久立伤骨 *Jiu li shang gu.*)

Prolonged standing may cause plantar fascitis which is experienced as heel or foot bone pain. Prolonged standing may also cause sacroiliac pain. Therefore, prolonged standing may damage the bones.

Prolonged movement damages the sinews. (久行伤筋 *Jiu xing shang jin.*)

The sinews gather at the joints and all movement occurs at the joints. Prolonged movement may damage the sinews, thus causing joint problems such as tennis elbow, carpal tunnel syndrome, and rotator cuff disorder. This is Chinese medicine's explanation of microtrauma due to repetitive strain.

Prolonged sitting damages the flesh. (久坐伤肉 *Jiu zuo shang rou.*)

The flesh is governed by the spleen according to five phase theory. Prolonged sitting damages the flesh by resulting in too much fat and not enough muscle. When sitting, the qi and blood are not stirred. Therefore, dampness and turbidity collect and accumulate, eventually congealing into phlegm or fat.

Sexual desire beyond measure mostly produces taxation detriment. (色欲过度，多成劳损。 *Se yu guo du, duo cheng lao sun.*)

According to Chinese medicine, too much sexual desire thus resulting in too much sexual activity damages and consumes the essence and qi. Therefore, it can result in taxation detriment, with "detriment" (损, *sun*) always implying vacuity.

[For] men, [it is] not ok not [to have] a woman. [For] women, [it is] not ok not [to have] a man. Not [having] a woman leads to desire stirring, [and] desire stirring leads to spirit taxation, [and] spirit taxation leads to detriment of long life. (男不可无女，女不可无男，无女则意动，意动则神劳，神劳则损寿。*Nan bu ke wu nu, nu bu ke wu nan, wu nu ze yi dong, yi dong ze shen lao, shen lao ze sun shou.*)

> According to this statement, it is not OK for men or women to go without sex. If one does, one's desire will stir which will, in turn, tax the spirit, and taxation of the spirit causes detriment to one's long life.

Food [and] drink, taxation [and] fatigue, joy [and] anger without discipline, [when they] initiate disease, [all have] heat within. (饮食，劳倦，喜怒不节，始病热中 *Yin shi, lao juan, xi nu be jie, shi bing re zhong.*)

> As this statement says, unregulated diet, unregulated physical activity, and unregulated psyche can all cause disease and can all especially cause heat evils within the body.

Phlegm
(痰, *tan*)

[If] fluids [and] humors contract disease, [they] transform into phlegm rheum. (津液受病，化为痰饮。*Jin ye shou bing, hua wei tan yin.*)

> Phlegm is nothing other than congealed dampness which, in turn, is nothing other than collected fluids and humors. Rheum is basically equivalent to dampness. Therefore, phlegm rheum is nothing other than diseased fluids and humors.

The root of phlegm is water dampness; if there is qi and fire, this leads to binding of phlegm. (痰本水湿，得气与火则结为痰 *Tan ben shui shi, de qi yu huo ze jie wei tan.*)

This statement likewise confirms that phlegm is nothing other than collected fluids which have transformed into dampness and congealed into phlegm. However, this statement goes on to say that qi and fire can cause the binding of phlegm. In this case, qi means qi stagnation and fire refers to the stewing and brewing of phlegm resulting in even more congelation.

Because phlegm is [essentially] water, its root is in the kidneys [and] its tip [or branch] is in the spleen. (盖痰即水也，其本在肾，其标在脾。 *Gai tan ji shui ye, qi ben zai shen, qi biao zai pi.*)
There are three viscera which control the movement of water fluids in the body, the lungs, spleen, and kidneys, with the spleen and kidneys being the two most important of these. Since phlegm is nothing other than congealed fluids, phlegm must be closely related to these three viscera. According to this statement, the root of phlegm is in the kidneys and its tip is in the spleen.

The spleen is the source of phlegm's engenderment. The lungs are the place where phlegm is stored. (脾为生痰之源，肺为所在痰藏。 *Pi wei sheng tan zhi yuan. Fei wei suo zai tan cang.*)
The previous statement not withstanding, this statement is more commonly quoted about the source of phlegm engenderment. Because the spleen governs water fluids and phlegm is congealed water fluids, dysfunction of the spleen is the source of phlegm engenderment. However, because the lungs often fill with phlegm when they are diseased, it is said that the lungs are the place where phlegm is stored.

Phlegm and rheum are not the same, phlegm [is] dense and rheum [is] thin, phlegm [is] turbid and rheum [is] clear. (痰与饮不同，痰浓而饮稀，痰浊而饮清。 *Tan yu yin bu tong, tan nong er yin xi, tan zhuo er yin qing.*)

Thickness [and] turbidity make for phlegm, clearness [and] thinness make for rheum. (稠浊者为痰，清稀者为饮。 *Chou zhuo zhe wei tan, qing xi zhe wei yin.*)

Phlegm [and] rheum are transformed from fluids [and] humors. Phlegm [is] turbid [and] rheum [is] clear. Phlegm is caused by fire, [and] rheum is caused by dampness. (痰饮皆津液所化，痰

浊饮清，痰因于火，饮因于湿也。*Tan yin jie jin ye suo hua, tan zhuo yin qing, tan yin yu huo, yin yin yu shi ye.*)

Rheum is due to rheum water not scattering and producing disease; phlegm is due to fire flaming, steaming, [and] burning and producing disease. Therefore, phlegm is thick [and] turbid, [and] rheum [is] clear [and] thin. (饮者，因饮水不散而成病；痰者，因火炎熏灼而成疾。故痰稠浊，饮清稀. *Yin zhe, yin yin shui bu san er cheng bing; tan zhe, yin huo yan xun zhuo er cheng yi. Gu tan chou zhuo; yin qing xi.*)

These four statements define the difference between phlegm and rheum. Phlegm is thick and turbid, while, comparatively, rheum is clear and thin. In point of fact, phlegm may be engendered without heat or fire.

[If] the three burners' qi [is] astringed [and] the vessel pathways [are] blocked [and] congested, water fluids [will] collect [and] gather [and do] not obtain diffusion [and] movement. [Such] gathering produces phlegm rheum. (三焦气涩，脉道闭塞，则水液停聚，不得宣行，聚成痰饮。*San jiao qi se, mai dao bi sai, ze shui ye ting ju, bu de xuan xing, ju cheng tan yin.*)

The passageways of the three burners are the pathways for the flow of water fluids in the body. This passage is, therefore, just another statement about how water fluids may collect and become dampness which then congeals to make phlegm.

Phlegm rheum [is] also a damp disease. (痰饮，湿病也。*Tan yin, shi bing ye.*)

Since phlegm rheum is created from dampness, it can be seen as a damp disease. In fact, in clinic, many of the same medicinals and acupoints are used to treat phlegm and dampness.

Phlegm [and] dampness lead to qi obstruction; qi obstruction leads to qi stagnation. (痰湿则气阻，气阻则气滞 *Tan shi ze qi zu, qi zu ze qi zhi.*)

This statement explains that both phlegm and dampness may lead to qi stagnation. This is because the phlegm and dampness obstruct and hinder the free flow of qi.

Without fire there is no engenderment of phlegm. (无火不生痰
Wu huo bu sheng tan.)

While the presence of fire certainly speeds and aggravates the engenderment of phlegm, in contemporary Chinese medicine we no longer take this saying as an absolute.

Phlegm congelation follows qi's upbearing and downbearing.
(痰凝随气升降 *Tan ning sui qi sheng jiang.*)

Once phlegm has been produced its movement in the body follows the movement of the qi. If the qi counterflows upward, so will phlegm. For instance, plum pit qi is a combination of phlegm and stagnant qi which have counterflowed upward to lodge in the throat. Similarly, mucus in the stools or abnormal vaginal discharge are often seen as phlegm which has descended to exit from the lower yin. In this case, phlegm descends because the spleen qi has failed to upbear this turbidity.

Strange diseases [are] mostly phlegm. (怪病多痰。 *Guai bing duo tan.*)

This saying can be interpreted in two ways. First, in strange diseases there is typically a lot of phlegm. Secondly, strange diseases are mostly due to phlegm. It all depends on how one translates the word 多 (*duo*). This word can either be translated as "mostly" or "a lot."

All [forms of] epilepsy [are due to] phlegm evils counterflowing upward. (癫痫者，痰邪逆上也。 *Dian xian zhe, tan xie ni shang ye.*)

According to this statement, all forms of epilepsy are complicated by at least some element of phlegm.

[In case of epilepsy, there] cannot not be phlegm drool blocking and congesting, misting and oppressing the cavities and orifices. (无非痰涎壅塞，迷闷孔窍。 *Wu fei tan xian yong sai, mi men kong qiao.*)

This statement likewise states that, if there is epilepsy, there must be phlegm misting the clear orifices above.

Phlegm existing in the lungs [it] leads to cough; in the stomach [it] leads to retching; in the head, [it] leads to dizziness; in the heart, [it] leads to palpitations; in the upper back, [it] leads to chill; [and] in the rib-sides, [it] leads to distention. (痰在肺则咳，在胃则呕，在头则眩，在心则悸，在背则冷，在胁则胀 *Tan zai fei ze ke, zai wei ze ou, zai tou ze xuan, zai xin ze ji, zai bei ze leng, zai xie ze zhang.*)

> This passage explains the common manifestations of phlegm in different parts of the body. In the lungs, phlegm causes coughing. In the stomach, it causing vomiting. In the head, it causes dizziness. In the heart, it causes palpitations. In the upper back, it causes chilling. This is because the phlegm obstructs the free flow and spreading of the yang qi. Therefore, in the absence of yang qi, there is chill. In the rib-side, it cause distention and fullness.

Phlegm follows fire's upbearing. (痰随火升 *Tan sui huo sheng.*)
> Fire often causes phlegm engendered in the middle burner to move upward to either the upper burner or head. In the upper burner, the phlegm may affect either the heart or lungs. In the head, it affects the clear orifices.

The source of hundreds of diseases is engendered by phlegm. (百病之源，皆生于痰。 *Bai bing zhi yuan, jie sheng yu tan.*)
> This saying states that phlegm either causes or complicates many, many diseases.

Fat people [have] lots of phlegm. (肥人多痰。 *Fei ren duo tan.*)

Fat people [have] lots of phlegm [and] therefore qi vacuity. Vacuity leads to the qi not moving. Therefore, phlegm is engendered. (肥人多痰，乃气虚也。虚则气不运行，故痰生之。 *Fei ren duo tan, nai qi xu ye. Xu ze qi bu yun xing, gu tan sheng zhi.*)
> Both of these statements say that fat people have lots of phlegm. However, the second says that it is qi vacuity which leads to this excess of phlegm. Because of qi vacuity, water fluids do not move but congeal into phlegm instead.

Phlegm [and] stasis [are] mutually involved. (痰瘀相关。 *Tan yu xiang guan.*)
> This statement can also be read either of two ways. The first is that blood stasis and phlegm are mutually related. In other words,

commonly, where there is one, there is the other. The second way of reading this saying is that phlegm and stasis mutually bar each other, which they do. The word 关 (*guan*) can either mean two things are related or that something is barred. For instance, to close or bar a door is 关门 (*guan men*). In this case, the presence of phlegm can block and obstruct the flow of blood, thus resulting in blood stasis, or the presence of blood stasis can hinder and obstruct the flow of water fluids, thus resulting in the engenderment of phlegm.

Blood Stasis
(血瘀, *xue yu*)

Stasis [is] accumulation of blood. (瘀，积血也。 *Yu, ji xue ye.*)
   According to this statement, blood stasis is the pathological accumulation of blood. However, within Chinese medicine, other synonyms for blood stasis are dead blood (死血, *si xue*), dry blood (干血, *gan xue*), and malign blood (恶血, *e xue*).

New diseases are in the channels; enduring diseases enter the network vessels. (新病在经，久病入络. *Xin bing zai jing, jiu bing ru luo.*)

[If] enduring disease is not cured, damage reaches the blood network vessels, the blood vessels do not flow smoothly, and [this] results in blood stasis. (久病不愈，伤及血络，血脉不畅，而致血瘀。 *Jiu bing bu yu, shang ji xue luo, xue mai bu chang, er zhi xue yu.*)
   The first of these two statements is by Ye Tian-shi. The second statement explains the clinical implications of Ye's statement.

[In] enduring diseases, there must be stasis. (久病必瘀. *Jiu bing bi yu.*)
   Later, Wang Qing-ren says essentially the same thing even more tersely. In enduring disease there must be blood stasis.

Enduring disease results in stasis. (久病从瘀。 *Jiu bing cong yu.*)
   Yet another statement that enduring diseases result in blood stasis. Therefore, it is extremely important to search for signs and symptoms in all enduring diseases.

[If] damp heat gathers and congests, the flow of the qi mechanism [will become] uneasy [and] the movement of blood will suffer obstruction resulting in the production of static blood. (湿热壅塞，气机不畅，血行受阻，致瘀血产生。*Shi re yong sai, qi ji bu chang, xue xing shou zu, zhi yu xue chan sheng.*)
This statement explains that damp heat may obstruct the flow of blood, thus causing blood stasis. In that case, there is both damp heat and blood stasis. Since the qi must also be depressed by these obstructions, this is frequently referred to as damp heat stasis and stagnation (湿热瘀滞, *shi re yu zhi*).

[If] warm qi is not moved, congealed blood brews and wraps and is not scattered, [the movement of] fluids and humors [is] rough [and they] seep [downward, if these] adhere and are not removed, various accumulations [will] be produced. (温气不行，凝血蕴裹而不散，津液涩渗，着而不去，而积皆成矣。*Wen qi bu xing, ning xue yun guo er bu san, jin ye se shen, zhuo er bu qu, er ji jie cheng yi.*)
This statement explains that heat may boil the blood until it congeals or becomes static. This obstructs the movement of fluids and humors, giving rise to dampness or phlegm. If these unite and are not removed, various types of masses may be produced within the body.

[If] blood contracts cold, it congeals [and] binds, [thus] producing lumps. [If] blood contracts heat, it boils [and] stews, [thus also] producing lumps. (血受寒则凝结成块，血受热则煎熬成块。*Xue shou han ze ning jie cheng kuai, xue shou re ze jian ao cheng kuai.*)
This statement explains how either heat or cold can form blood stasis which can then form masses within the body.

Qi is formless [and therefore] is not able to bind [into] lumps. Bound lumps all must have the form of blood. (气无形不能结块，结块者必有形之血也。*Qi wu xing bu neng jie kuai, jie kuai zhe bing you xing zhi xue ye.*)
This statement explains that qi is formless and, therefore, cannot be directly responsible for lumps or masses in the body which have form or physical substance. Blood on the other hand is a substance

and does have form. Therefore, it is the binding of blood or blood stasis which creates masses in the body.

Disease Mechanisms
(病机, *bing ji*)

Disease mechanisms are the dynamic effects once disease causes set a pathological train in motion. The more one understands disease mechanisms, the easier it is to accurately and efficiently discriminate patterns. Unfortunately, many textbooks on basic Chinese medical theory give relatively a lot of attention to disease causes but scanty attention to disease mechanisms. Most commonly, lengthy discussions of disease mechanisms are found in clinical manuals, not introductory textbooks, or in the commentary sections of clinical trials and case histories. Below, I have divided commonly repeated statements about disease mechanisms into a number of different categories in order to make referencing such statements easier.

Yin-Yang Disease Mechanisms
(阴阳病机, *yin yang bing ji*)

Some of these statements appear under the introductory section on yin and yang. However, they are repeated here and explained specifically in terms of human pathophysiology.

Detriment of yang affects yin. (阳损及阴 *Yang sun ji yin.*)
While "detriment" is often used as a synonym of "damage" or part of the compound term "detriment [and] damage (损伤, *sun shang*)," it always means damage resulting in vacuity, not repletion. Therefore, this statement means that yang vacuity may eventually result in yin vacuity as well.

Detriment to yin affects yang. (阴损及阳 *Yin sun ji yang.*)
Based on the above explanation, this statement means that yin vacuity will eventually result in yang vacuity as well.

[If] yang [becomes] vacuous, yin [becomes] exuberant. (阳虚阴盛 *Yang xu yin sheng.*)

According to this statement, if yang becomes vacuous and, therefore, is not able to move and transform yin, then yin will become exuberant or replete. However, this does not mean that righteous yin becomes replete but rather that yin evils, such as cold, dampness, and phlegm, will become replete.

[If] yin [becomes] exuberant, yang [becomes] debilitated. (阴盛阳衰 *Yin sheng yang shuai.*)

Similarly, in this case, yin exuberance refers to yin evil repletions, such as cold, dampness, and phlegm. If these hinder and obstruct the movement and transformation of yang qi within the body, yang qi will suffer damage and become debilitated or vacuous.

[If] yang [becomes] vacuous, water spills over. (阳虚水泛 *Yang xu shui fan.*)

This statement is a corollary of the above. If yang qi becomes too vacuous to move and transform water fluids in the body, these fluids will accumulate and may spill over. In particular, when water spills over, it mostly moves out of the middle burner and into the lower burner or into the spaces between the skin and flesh, as in edema.

Yang exuberance damages yin. (阳盛阴伤 *Yang sheng yin shang.*)

If yang become hyperactive, it engenders heat or fire and this heat or fire may damage yin, leading to yin vacuity.

[If] yin [becomes] vacuous, yang [becomes] hyperactive. (阴虚阳亢 *Yin xu yang kang.*)

Because yin is the root of yang, yin vacuity failing to control yang may lead to yang hyperactivity and the engenderment of heat.

[If] yin [becomes] vacuous, yang floats. (阴虚阳浮 *Yin xu yang fu.*)

This statement is a corollary of the above. If yin becomes vacuous and insufficient and is unable to control yang, yang may float upward in the body to accumulate in the heart and lungs or to harass the clear orifices above.

[If] yin [becomes] vacuous, fire [becomes] effulgent. (阴虚火旺 *Yin xu huo wang.*)

If yin becomes so vacuous as to lose control over yang, heat is engendered. If this heat is virulent enough, it will manifest as fire effulgence, an even hotter form of heat.

Prevalence of yang leads to heat. (阳胜则热 *Yang sheng ze re.*)

Because yang in the body is heat, prevalence of yang means that there will also be a lot of heat.

Prevalence of yin leads to cold. (阴胜则寒 *Yin sheng ze han.*)

Prevalence of yin in the body mostly means cold and/or dampness. Obviously, cold leads to cold. However, dampness may also lead to cold. If dampness damages the spleen and kidneys, then there will be a lack of yang qi in the body, and a lack of yang qi means a lack of warmth and, therefore, the presence of cold.

Yin evils damage yang; yang evils damage yin. (阴邪伤阳，阳邪伤阴 *Yin xie shang yang, yang xie shang yin.*)

Here, yin evils damaging yang refer to a prevalence of yin as explained above, while yang evils damaging yin refer to a prevalence of yang evils also explained above.

Yin vacuity leads to internal heat. (阴虚则内热 *Yin xu ze nei re.*)

As stated above, yin vacuity failing to control yang typically leads to the engenderment of heat or fire. However, this heat is internally engendered heat. Therefore, yin vacuity leads to internal heat.

Yang vacuity leads to external cold. (阳虚则外寒 *Yang xu ze wai han.*)

Yang vacuity is usually associated with a lack of defensive qi. In that case, external cold evils may easily invade the body leading to externally contracted cold.

[If] yang [becomes] vacuous, heat is emitted [*i.e.,* there is fever]. (阳虚发热 *Yang xu fa re.*)

At first sight, this statement seems contradictory. However, if yang becomes vacuous and loses its root, what is left of the yang qi may float upward and outward, thus effusing and emitting. Hence, what yang remains is experienced in the upper and exterior parts of the body.

[If] yin [becomes] exhausted, yang deserts. (阴竭阳脱 *Yin jie yang tuo.*)

If yin becomes completely exhausted, yang deserts by floating upward and outward, effusing and being emitted from the pores. If there is yang desertion, there is spontaneous sweating with prostration and syncope.

Vacuous yang floats upward. (阳虚上浮 *Yang xu shang fu.*)

As explained above, vacuous yang having lost its root in its lower source may float upward and outward in the body. If so, it will manifest signs and symptoms of heat above (上热, *shang re*) and cold below (下寒, *xia han*).

Profuse sweating damages yin. (汗多伤阴 *Han duo shang yin.*)

Enduring dysentery damages yin. (痢久伤阴 *Li jiu shang yin.*)

Because all the yin fluids in the body share a common source and are mutually connected, any loss of fluids, whether by profuse sweating, enduring dysentery, etc. may damage yin and lead to yin vacuity.

[If] yang vacuity heat encroaches above, [there is] yin vacuity [and] essence decline below. (阳虚热冒于上，阴虚精遗于下 *Yang xu re mao yu shang, yin xu jing yi yu xia.*)

This is because yin vacuity below (*i.e.,* kidney yin vacuity) is failing to control yang which then ascends, encroaching on the organs and tissues of the upper body.

[If] yang is vacuous, qi [may] not contain the blood. (阳虚气不摄血 *Yang xu qi bu she xue.*)

Within the human body, yang simply refers to enough of an accumulation of qi in one place for there to be warmth as well as function. Therefore, all yang vacuity includes qi vacuity even though the word qi may not be present. Since one of the functions of the qi is to contain the blood within its vessels, yang vacuity may lead to qi not containing the blood and hence pathological bleeding.

[If] yin is vacuous, ministerial fire [may] move frenetically [and] force the blood to overflow outside. (阴虚相火妄动，逼血外溢 *Yin xu xiang huo wang dong, bi xue wai yi.*)

As we have seen above, if yin is vacuous, yang may become hyperactive. Ministerial fire is the fire of the life-gate which connects upward to the heart. If yin fails to control yang, ministerial fire may stir frenetically. In this case, because of the close connection between ministerial fire and the liver, heat may enter the blood aspect. If this heat then causes the blood to stir frenetically outside its pathways, bleeding will occur.

Yang disease erupts in winter; yin disease erupts in summer. (阳病发于冬，阴病发于夏 *Yang bing fa yu dong, yin bing fa yu xia.*)

This statement may be interpreted in either of two ways. The first is the more straightforward. In that case, yang disease refers to yang vacuity. Since winter is the time when yang is most necessary to keep the body warm, yang disease erupts in winter. Likewise, since summer is the hottest time of the year and heat may damage yin, yin disease, meaning disease due to yin vacuity, erupts in summer. However, there is another way to interpret this statement. In winter, the weather is cold and this causes constriction of the exterior. This in turn results in heat being trapped in the interior of the body. Because this is depressed internally, yang disease erupts in winter. In summer, the weather is hot and people often eat and drink too many chilled, uncooked foods. This may damage the spleen and lead to accumulation of yin dampness. Therefore, yin disease erupts in summer.

Yang vacuity leads to qi stagnation, and qi stagnation leads to inability to lead the blood to gather in the channels. (阳虚则气滞，气滞则不能导血归经 *Yang xu ze qi zhi, qi zhi ze bu neng dao xue gui jing.*)

Yang vacuity means that there is insufficient qi to stir or move as well as vacuity cold causing constriction and tension. Thus yang vacuity leads to qi stagnation. However, qi stagnation may lead to the engenderment of blood stasis, and this stasis may force the blood to move outside its pathways, thus causing bleeding.

Great sweating, accumulation, and overtaxation can all damage yang. (大汗积劳都是伤阳 *Da han ji lao dou shi shang yang.*)

When we sweat, we always lose some yang qi in the process, since it is the yang qi which moves sweat out of the body. Therefore, great sweating can damage yang. Accumulation means accumulations of evil qi in the abdomen. Such accumulations hinder and obstruct the free flow of the visceral qi, leading to their dysfunction. Since the viscera engender and transform the qi, such damage to visceral function may eventually lead to an insufficiency of yang qi. Overtaxation directly consumes the qi. Overtaxation means nothing other than excessive function, be it physical, verbal, mental, or sexual. Since yang is nothing other than qi, overtaxation may damage yang.

[If there is] yang vacuity, heat will encroach above. (阳虚冒热于上 *Yang xu mao re yu shang.*)

Here again we are talking about upwardly floating yang due to vacuous yang's having lost its root in the lower burner.

[If there is] yin vacuity, [there will be] essence efflux from below. (阴虚精遗于下 *Yin xu jing yi yu xia.*)

Essence efflux refers to involuntary seminal emission. When there is yin vacuity, there is also some element of qi vacuity as well. If the qi does not secure and astringe the essence, if may efflux. In addition, when there is yin vacuity, ministerial fire tends to become hyperactive, and the heat of stirring ministerial fire may also force the essence out of the body involuntarily.

[If] yin is depleted below, yang [will] float upward. (阴亏于下，阳浮于上 *Yin kui yu xia, yang fu yu shang.*)

This is yet another expression of yin vacuity failing to control yang which then ascends above.

Enduring diarrhea [and] enduring dysentery both can damage yin and can also damage yang. (久泻久痢，既能伤阴，亦能伤阳 *Jiu xie jiu li, ji neng shang yin, yi neng shang yang.*)

Because of the loss of fluids caused by enduring diarrhea or dysentery, there obviously may be damage to yin. However, because yin and yang are mutually rooted, yin vacuity may eventually lead to yang vacuity as well. In addition, each time we defecate, we lose some yang qi, since it is the qi which moves the feces out of the body. Therefore, excessive defecation may also result in a direct loss of yang qi.

[If there is] a surplus of yin, [there will be] profuse sweating [and] bodily cold. (阴气有余为多汗身寒 *Yin qi you yu wei duo han shen han.*)

Here, a surplus of yin refers to cold and damp evils, whether externally contracted or internally engendered. Because these may damage the spleen and lead to qi vacuity, qi may be too weak to contain the sweat within the body. Thus there is profuse sweating. On the other hand, because there may not be enough yang qi to warm the body properly, there may be bodily cold.

If the upper back detests cold, there is yang insufficiency. (背恶 寒者阳不足也 *Bei e han zhe yang bu zu ye.*)

The upper back is a place in the body where all the yang qi unites. Therefore, if specifically the upper body is cold, this may indicate that the yang qi is vacuous and insufficient.

[If] the body is habitually yin vacuous, dampness will transform into heat. (素体阴虚，湿从热化 *Su ti yin xu, shi cong re hua.*)

Habitual yin vacuity will give rise to vacuity heat. If there is dampness in the body, this heat will combine with this dampness to produce damp heat.

Yang vacuity leads to fright palpitations; yin vacuity leads to vexation. (阳虚则悸，阴虚则烦 *Yang xu ze ji, yin xu ze fan.*)

Yang vacuity again means that there is insufficient qi. If there is specifically insufficient yang qi to warm and move the heart, then there may be palpitations. Vexation refers to an annoying dry heat sensation in the middle of the chest. If yin vacuity gives rise to vacuity heat or fire effulgence, this heat may float upward to accumulate in the chest, thus producing vexation.

[If] yin vacuity endures for days, [one] must see qi vacuity. (阴 虚日久，必见气虚. *Yin xu ri jiu, bi jian qi xu.*)

The existence of yin is necessary for yang to function. Therefore, yin vacuity eventually leads to qi vacuity.

[By] 40 years [of age], yin qi [is] automatically half. (年四十，阴气自半 *Nian si shi, yin qi zi ban.*)

According to the *Nei Jing (Inner Classic)*, by 40 years of age, yin has been half consumed by the activities of living. This is why, in clinic, we mostly see signs and symptoms of yin vacuity after 40 years of age. This is, of course, unless there is a former heaven natural endowment insufficiency of yin or unusual consumption of yin by such extreme activities as drug abuse.

[If] yang qi declines day [by day], detriment arrives day [by day]. (阳气日衰，损于日至。 *Yang qi ri shuai, sun yu ri zhi.*)

According to this statement, if yang qi declines day by day, then one suffers detriment also day by day. This statement mostly has to do with the yang qi decline associated with aging. Therefore, one could gloss this statement that, if yang qi declines day by day, one gets more and more senile (in the large sense of that word) also day by day.

Five Phase Disease Mechanisms
(五行病机, *wu xing bing ji*)

Water depleted at its origin leads to yin vacuity disease with repeated exiting. (水亏其源则阴虚之病叠出 *Shui kui qi yuan ze yin xu zhi bing die chu.*)

The origin of water in the human body is the kidneys, the root of true yin. So water depleted at its origin refers to kidney yin vacuity. As this statement says, kidney yin vacuity leads to yin vacuity disease of any of the other viscera and bowels as well as along with repeated exiting. Here, repeated exiting refers to polyuria, nocturia, and seminal emission, any and all of which may be associated with kidney yin vacuity.

Fire debilitated at its root leads to yang vacuity disease with repeated arising. (火衰其本则阳虚病叠生 *Huo shuai qi ben ze yang xu bing die sheng.*)

Likewise, the root of fire in the human body is the kidneys, the root of true yang. Therefore, kidney yang vacuity leads to yang vacuity of other viscera as well. In this case, rootless yang may ascend or float upward, thus resulting in "repeated arising."

[If] fire counterflows [and] qi ascends, the throat [will be] inhibited. (火逆上气，咽喉不利。 *Huo ni shang qi, yan hou bu li.*)

This statement is not necessarily speaking about the fire phase. However, since it begins with the word "fire," it has been placed in this category of disease mechanisms. In fact, this fire is any internally engendered fire but usually depressive fire. If such depressive fire and counterflowing qi ascend, they often become trapped or accumulate in the throat. This is because the throat is narrow and is like a bottleneck. If heat and counterflowing qi lodge in the throat, the free flow of the throat qi will be inhibited and sore throat typically occurs.

Qi & Blood Disease Mechanisms
(气血病机, *qi xue bing ji*)

Qi [and] blood may lose their normalcy. (气血失常。*Qi xue shi chang*.)
Qi and blood may lose their constancy or normalcy. Mostly this means the constancy or normalcy of their flow through the channels and vessels. Both qi and blood must flow in order to be healthy and well.

The qi mechanism [or dynamic] may lose its regulation. (气机失调。*Qi ji shi tiao*.)
The qi mechanism governs the upbearing and downbearing, exiting and entering of the qi. If the qi mechanism loses its regulation, the four movements of the qi will not be normal.

The qi mechanism [may become] depressed [and] stagnant. (气机郁滞。*Qi ji yu zhi*.)
This means that the flow of the qi mechanism may be inhibited and lose its free flow.

The upper qi may be insufficient. (上气不足。*Shang qi bu zu*.)
The upper qi means the upper burner qi or the heart-lung qi. In this case, the heart and/or lung qi are insufficient.

The central qi may fall downward. (中气下陷。*Zhong qi xia xian*.)
This means that vacuous spleen or central qi may fall downward to the lower burner resulting in various types of prolapse.

[If] yang qi does not arrive at the outside, then water dampness will forcibly occupy its place. (阳气不到之外， 即是水湿盘踞 之所 *Yang qi bu dao zhi wai, ji shi shui shi pan ju zhi suo.*)

If, due to vacuity, yang qi does not move water fluids through the exterior, fluids will collect and transform into damp evils.

[If] yang qi is faint, the upper back [will be] cold [and] the feet frigid. (阳气是微，则背寒足冷 *Yang qi shi wei, ze bei han zu leng.*)

As we have seen above, the upper back is a meeting place of all yang in the body. Similarly, cold feet are symptoms of kidney yang vacuity failing to descend and warm the feet. Therefore, upper back cold and cold feet are symptoms of yang vacuity.

[If] yang qi has a surplus, the constructive qi will not move and will eventually erupt into welling and flat abscesses. (阳气有 余，营气不行，乃发为痈疽 *Yang qi you yu, ying qi bu xing, nai fa wei yong ju.*)

If yang qi has a surplus, it will typically float upward and outward to congest with the exterior where it will hamper and obstruct the free flow of the constructive qi. Instead, the heat associated with a surplus of yang will boil and stew the constructive and blood causing them to erupt into welling and flat abscesses.

[If] yang qi is vacuous, [it will be] unable to engender [and] transform fluids [and] humors, resulting in a thirsty mouth. (阳气虚，不能升化津液，故口渴 *Yang qi xu, bu neng sheng hua jin ye, gu kou ke.*)

One of the functions of yang qi is to move water fluids throughout the body so that they can moisten and sprinkle all the tissues of the body. If yang qi is vacuous, it may not be strong enough to move water fluids upward to the mouth. In that case, the mouth will be deprived of moistening and will be dry instead. Thus there will be thirst inside the mouth.

Qi vacuity leads to fatigue [and] lack of strength. (气虚则怠无 力 *Qi xu ze dai wu li.*)

Fatigue is, ipso facto, a symptom of qi vacuity. In fact, it is one of the most important symptoms of qi vacuity. It is also the qi which empowers the strength of the body and extremities. Therefore, qi vacuity leads to fatigue and lack of strength.

Blood debility leads to the liver not being nourished. (血亏则肝 无所养 *Xue kui ze gan wu suo yang.*)

The liver stores the blood. Therefore, the liver has an especially close relationship with the blood. Further, the blood nourishes the liver just as it does all the other organs and tissues of the body. Since blood debility is a synonym for blood vacuity, blood vacuity may lead to the liver being malnourished.

[If there is] blood vacuity of the body, liver yang easily upbears. (血虚之体，肝阳易升 *Xue xu zhi ti, gan yang yi sheng.*)

Here, the word "body" refers to the substance of the liver. Thus blood vacuity of the body means a liver blood vacuity. Since blood and essence share a common source and the liver commonly has a surplus, liver blood vacuity may lead to kidney yin vacuity with yin failing to control yang. In that case, liver yang may easily become hyperactive and ascend.

Qi stagnation leads to blood stasis. (气滞则血瘀 *Qi zhi ze xue yu.*)

Since the qi moves the blood, if the qi stops, the blood will also typically stop. Hence qi stagnation leads to blood stasis.

Qi depression leads to glomus [and] oppression. (气郁则痞闷 *Qi yu ze pi men.*)

Glomus is a feeling as if there were a lump in the abdomen. However, when palpated, there is no lump. Oppression means chest oppression, a feeling of fullness in the chest, while qi depression is another term for qi stagnation. If the qi is stagnant and depressed and does not flow freely through the abdomen and chest, it may accumulate giving rise to feelings of glomus and oppression.

Blood vacuity leads to forgetfulness. (血虚则发落 *Xue xu ze fa luo.*)

The blood nourishes the heart spirit, and memory is associated with the function of the spirit. Therefore, blood vacuity may lead to forgetfulness. In point of fact, forgetfulness most commonly indicates a heart-spleen dual vacuity.

Blood not returning to the liver leads to [one] not [being able] to lie down [*i.e.* to sleep]. (血不归肝则不卧 *Xue bu gui gan ze bu wo.*)

When we lie down and sleep, the blood returns to be stored in the liver. Since sleep is nothing other than the yang qi sinking down and within yin-blood, if the blood does not return to the liver, this can be a cause of insomnia.

Qi stagnation leads to tenseness [*i.e.* cramping] internally. (气滞则里急 *Qi zhi ze li ji.*)

This statement equates tension or cramping with qi stagnation. In this case, we can say that cramping is one of the subjective sensations of the qi not flowing freely and smoothly.

Qi stagnation [may lead to] blood stasis. (气滞血瘀。*Qi zhi xue yu.*)

Because qi moves the blood, qi stagnation may lead to blood stasis.

Qi vacuity [may lead to] blood stasis. (气虚血瘀。*Qi xu xue yu.*)
Likewise, if qi is vacuous and weak and lacks the strength or power to move the blood, the blood can become static.

Qi vacuity engenders phlegm; blood stagnation turns into stasis. (气虚生痰，血滞成淤 *Qi xu sheng tan, xue zhi cheng yu.*)

If qi is too vacuous to move and transform water fluids, fluids collect and transform into dampness, while if dampness endures, it congeals into phlegm. Normally, the term blood stagnation is a lesser used synonym for blood stasis. But here, it says that blood stagnation turns into stasis, thus suggesting that stagnation is not the same as stasis. One way of interpreting this is that, if the qi within the blood becomes stagnant, the blood becomes static.

Hundreds of diseases are mostly engendered by the qi; exterior vacuity is qi scattering and internal stagnation is qi obstruction. (百病多生于气，表虚为气散，里滞为气阻 *Bai bing duo sheng yu qi, biao xu wei qi san, li zhi wei qi zu.*)

This statement says that many, many diseases are caused by diseases of the qi. The statement then goes on to give two examples of qi disease. If the qi in the exterior is vacuous, the defensive exterior is scattered or dispersed. If the qi in the interior is stagnant, then there is qi obstruction.

Qi weakness leads to drink [and] food brewing into phlegm. (气
弱则饮食酿痰 *Qi ruo ze yin shi niang tan.*)

If the qi is too vacuous and weak to move and transform food and
drink, this turbidity may collect and accumulate to eventually
congeal into phlegm.

Qi dryness leads to the clear orifices not being disinhibited. (气
燥则清窍不利 *Qi zao ze qing qiao bu li.*)

In order for any tissue or organ to function normally, it must receive
enough water fluids to moisten it. However, it is the qi which moves
water fluids throughout the body. Therefore, if the qi is so dry that
fluids cannot moisten the clear orifices in the upper body, they will be
inhibited and won't connect freely with the outside world.

All diseases [are] mostly engendered by depression. (诸病多生
于郁 *Zhu bing duo sheng yu yu.*)

"Depression" here may mean any of the six depressions (六郁, *liu
yu*). The six depressions are qi (气, *qi*), blood (血, *xue*), dampness
(湿, *shi*), phlegm (痰, *tan*), food (食, *shi*), and fire (火, *huo*). However,
of the six depressions, qi depression or stagnation is the most
common and can lead to or aggravate any of the other five.
Therefore, it is rare to find a disease which does not include some
element of depression.

All itching is vacuity; it is blood not constructing. (诸痒为虚，
血不荣也 *Zhu yang wei xu, xue bu rong ye.*)

According to this statement, all itching is due to blood vacuity not
constructing and nourishing the qi within the skin. Because there is a
lack of blood to mother the qi, the qi moves frenetically throughout
the skin and this is subjectively experienced as itching.

Qi vacuity leads to inability to engender [and] transform fluids
and humors. (气虚则不能生化津液 *Qi xu ze bu neng sheng hua
jin ye.*)

Fluids and humors in the body are engendered and transformed by
the spleen qi from the food and drink taken in by the stomach.
Therefore, qi vacuity leads to the inability to engender and
transform fluids and humors.

Qi vacuity leads to urination being frequent; yin vacuity leads to urination being difficult. (气虚则小便数，阴虚则小便难 *Qi xu ze xiao bian shu, yin xu ze xiao bian nan.*)

Qi vacuity leads to an inability to contain water fluids within the body. Therefore, urination is frequent. As for the second half of this statement, there are two ways to interpret it. First, yin's enrichment and moistening are necessary for all tissues and organs to function normally. Therefore, yin vacuity leads to an inability of the bladder to function properly. Since its function is to store and discharge fluids from the body, urination is difficult. Secondly, yin vacuity may simply lead to scanty urine. Thus urination is difficult because there is not the urine to discharge.

Blood vacuity leads to numbness. (血虚则麻 *Xue xu ze ma.*)

Blood nourishes the skin, and one of the functions of the skin is sensitivity. Therefore, if the blood is too vacuous to nourish the skin, there may be insensitivity or numbness.

Blood vacuity leads to liver dryness, [and] liver dryness leads to lots of anger [and] lots of fright. (血虚则肝燥，肝燥则多怒多惊 *Xue xu ze gan zao, gan zao ze duo nu duo jing.*)

Anger is the subjective experience of liver depression. Since the liver qi can only function if it receives adequate blood to nourish it, blood vacuity leading to liver dryness also leads to excessive anger. Because bile was associated with courage in ancient China and the liver secretes bile which is then stored in the gallbladder, blood vacuity failing to nourish the liver may also lead to excessive fright if we posit that excessive fright is the absence of courage.

[If] blood [and] qi bind and gather [and] cannot resolve [and] scatter, their poison is like gu. (血气结聚，不可解散，其毒如蛊 *Xue qi jie ju, bu ke jie san, qi du ru gu.*)

Gu refers to an invisible type of worms or parasites which cause very complicated, multisystem conditions. Therefore, this statement is saying that unresolved qi stagnation and blood stasis likewise cause complicated, multisystem diseases.

[If there is] free flow, there is no pain; [if there is] pain there is lack of free flow. 通则不痛；不通则通. *Tong ze bu tong; bu tong ze tong.*)

If qi and blood are not harmonious within the vessels and network vessels, there is pain. (脉络中气血不和则痛 *Mai luo zhong qi xue bu he ze tong.*)

> Both these statements say essentially the same thing. If there is free flow of the qi and blood within the channels and vessels, then there is no pain. However, if there is pain, then that is nothing other than a lack of free flow of the qi and blood within the channels and network vessels.

Blood vacuity leads to network vessel pain. (血虚则络痛 *Xue xu ze luo tong.*)

> As we have seen above, the network vessels are said to be full of blood. If there is a network vessel blood vacuity, then the network vessels cannot perform their function. Their function is to promote the flow of qi and blood. Because there is a lack of free flow, there is pain.

Blood vacuity leads to wind stirring. (血虚则风动 *Xue xu ze feng dong.*)

> Internally engendered wind is nothing other than pathologically stirring qi. Because the blood is the mother and root of the qi, blood vacuity may lead to qi moving frenetically and chaotically in the body. Thus blood vacuity leads to wind stirring.

[If] the constructive qi is insufficient, the facial color is blue-green. (营气不足面色青 *Ying qi bu zu mian se qing.*)

> According to this statement, if the constructive qi is vacuous or insufficient, the facial complexion is blue-green or cyanotic.

[If] the defensive qi is insufficient, the facial color is yellow. (卫气不足面色黄 *Wei qi bu zu mian se huang.*)

> On the other hand, if the defensive qi is vacuous and insufficient, the facial complexion is yellow.

Constructive vacuity gives rise to heat; defensive vacuity gives rise to cold. (营虚生热; 卫虚生寒. *Ying xu sheng re; Wei xu sheng han.*)

> For the purposes of this statement, constructive vacuity is related to a blood and yin vacuity. In that case, yin fails to control yang which becomes hyperactive and engenders heat. Similarly, for the purposes of this statement, defensive vacuity is related to yang

vacuity, and, since yang is inherently warm, lack of yang leads to the presence of cold.

Constructive [qi] vacuity leads to insensitivity; defensive qi vacuity leads to lack of use. (营虚则不仁; 卫气虚则不用. *Ying xu ze bu ren; Wei qi xu ze bu yong.*)

In this dichotomy, insensitivity (不仁, *bur en*) is juxtaposed with lack of use (不用, *bu yong*). "Use" always implies yang qi, while insensitivity usually implies the function of the skin as nourished by blood. Therefore, once again, the constructive qi is linked to the blood, while the defensive qi is linked to the yang qi.

Astringency and non-movement of the defensive qi leads to insensitivity. (卫气涩而不行则不仁 *Wei qi se er bu xing ze bu ren.*)

Astringency means constriction which then leads to non-movement. In this case, non-movement of the defensive qi is posited as the reason for the insensitivity of the skin.

Scanty blood [and] qi pertain to the heart. (血气少者属于心 *Xue qi shao zhe shu yu xin.*)

Scanty qi and blood mean blood vacuity. Why qi and blood vacuity is said here to pertain to the heart is that the heart spirit is constructed out of the qi which is nourished by the blood. Therefore, any qi and blood vacuity is likely to have some adverse affect on the function of the heart.

[If] blood stasis is not eliminated, new blood is not engendered. (淤血不去，则新血不生 *Yu xue bu qu, ze xin xue bu sheng.*)

This is an extremely important statement. It means that blood stasis hinders the creation of new or fresh blood. Therefore, most blood stasis eventually becomes complicated by blood vacuity. In addition, if there is blood vacuity and one does not simultaneously address the presence of any stasis, treatment for supplementing the blood will not be effective.

[If there is] debility and detriment of qi and blood, the interstices will not be secured and external wind may cause movement of internal wind. (气血亏损，腠理不固，外风因动内风 *Qi xue kui sun, cou li bu gu, wai feng yin dong nei feng.*

According to this statement, if there is qi and blood vacuity, the defensive exterior may be left unsecured and wind evils may enter the body. However, once in the body, external wind evils may stir and aggravate any tendency to internal wind.

If the constructive and blood are debilitated and consumed, they will not be able to construct and nourish the channels and vessels. (营血亏耗，不能营养经脉 *Ying xue kui hao, bun eng ying yang jing mai.*)

Here again, the constructive is linked to the blood and both the constructive and blood are said to construct and nourish the channels and vessels. Without this construction and nourishment, the channels and vessels cannot perform their function.

Essence-blood insufficiency leads to fear. (精血不足则恐 *Jing xue bu zu ze kong.*)

This statement can be explained in two ways. First, the linking of the essence and blood implies the liver and kidneys. "Essence and blood [share] a common source; the liver and kidneys [share] a common source." Thus it is a liver-kidney dual vacuity that leads to fear. In the case of the liver, liver vacuity leads to an absence of courage, while, in the case of the kidneys, fear is the affect of the kidneys. On the other hand, if there is heart spirit, there is courage, and the spirit is nourished by essence and blood. Either way one looks at it, essence and blood vacuity lead to fear. Interestingly, many pervasive developmental disorders are clinically associated with timidity and fearfulness.

Removal of blood leads to yin debility and fire effulgence; fire effulgence leads to hidden movement of liver wind. (血去则阴亏火旺，火旺则肝风暗动 *Xue qu ze yin kui huo wang, huo wang ze gan feng an dong.*)

In this statement, removal of blood may simply refer to bleeding, in which case, excessive bleeding may lead to yin vacuity failing to control yang. In that case, yang hyperactivity may engender heat or fire effulgence, and fire effulgence may stir any tendency to liver wind. However, the removal of blood may also refer to dispelling of stasis which is an attacking, draining therapy. When used inappropriately or excessively, it too can damage yin, leading to yang hyperactivity, etc.

Qi [and] blood insufficiency leads to feeling cold. (气血不足则
觉寒 *Qi xue bu zu ze jue han.*)
> Qi and blood vacuity may lead to cold because qi is inherently
> warm. Ipso facto, an absence of warmth produces a feeling of cold.
> Then why include blood in this statement? This is because blood is
> the mother of qi, and a pure qi vacuity is rarely seen in clinic.
> Where there is one, there is typically at least some element of the
> other.

Surplus of blood leads to anger, insufficiency to fear. (血有余则
怒，不足则恐 *Xue you yu ze nu, bu zu ze kong.*)
> Surplus of blood refers in this case to blood stasis, and static blood
> impedes the free flow of the qi. Hence static blood is rarely not
> complicated by liver depression, and anger is the subjective
> experience of liver depression qi stagnation. As we have seen
> above, blood vacuity may cause fear since blood is not nourishing
> the heart spirit.

Surplus of qi leads to panting, cough, and upward qi; insufficiency leads to uninhibited breathing [but] shortness of qi [*i.e.,*
breath]. (气有余则喘咳上气，不足则息利少气 *Qi you yu ze
chuan ke shang qi, bu zu ze xi li shao qi.*)
> Surplus of qi in this case refers to evil qi lodged in the lungs which
> then hinders the diffusion and downbearing of the lung qi. This
> causes panting and coughing, both species of upward counterflow
> of the lung qi. Insufficient lung qi leads to uninhibited inhalation and
> exhalation but shortness of breath.

Qi depression engenders phlegm; blood vacuity engenders wind.
(气郁生痰，血虚生风 *Qi yu sheng tan, xue xu sheng feng.*)
> As we have seen above, qi vacuity failing to move and transform
> water fluids can lead to phlegm engenderment. However, if blood is
> vacuous, it may fail to mother and root the qi. Instead, the qi moves
> frenetically. This is the same thing as stirring wind. Thus, blood
> vacuity engenders internal wind.

Insufficiency of blood leads to dry, constipated stools. (血不足
则大便燥而秘 *Xue bu zu ze da bian zao er bi.*)
> As we have seen above, blood and fluids share a common source.
> Thus, blood vacuity may lead to fluid dryness of the large intestine.

In that case, there is insufficient blood and fluids to "float the boat." Instead, the stools are dry and bound or constipated.

Depression and binding lead to gathering of fire, and fire leads to damage of the fluids. (郁结则聚火，火则伤津 *Yu jie ze ju huo, huo ze shang jin.*)
Depression here refers primarily to qi depression transforming heat or fire. Fire then may go on to damage fluids, giving rise to dryness and yin vacuity.

Qi depression transforms fire; fire depression engenders phlegm. (气郁化火，火郁生痰 *Qi yu hua huo, huo yu sheng tan.*)
Similar to the foregoing statement, qi depression may engender fire. Then, a mixture of fire and qi stagnation easily engenders phlegm. The fire boils the fluids which congeal into phlegm, while the qi stagnation prevents fluids from moving. Instead they collect and congeal into phlegm.

Depression damages the liver, [while] food damages the stomach. (郁伤肝，食伤胃。 *Yu shang gan, shi shang wei.*)
This statement refers again to qi depression. Qi depression causes liver depression qi stagnation. It is food depression or food stagnation which damages the stomach.

Qi repletion is heat; qi vacuity is cold. (气实者，热也；气虚者，寒也。 *Qi shi zhe, re ye; qi xu zhe, han ye.*)

[If] qi having a surplus promotes the existence of fire, insufficiency leads to the promotion of the presence of cold. (气有余便是火，不足则便是寒 *Qi you yu bian shi huo, bu zu ze bian shi han.*)
Because qi is yang and inherently warm, lots of qi means there is lots of warmth. Therefore, it is easy for fire to be transformed from this heat. Conversely, insufficient qi means a lack of warmth and the presence of cold.

Blood follows qi's fall. (血随气陷 *Xue sui qi xian.*)
Because qi moves the blood, if qi falls downward in the body, blood typically follows suit. In that case, there will be bleeding hemorrhoids, hemafecia, hematuria, and meno- and/or metrorrhagia.

Qi follows blood's desertion. (气随血脱。 *Qi sui xue tuo.*)
Because blood is the mother of the qi, if blood deserts due to massive hemorrhage, this will also lead to qi desertion with prostration, syncope, and spontaneous perspiration.

Blood contracting heat leads to boiling [and] stewing producing lumps. (血受热则煎熬成块. *Xue shou re ze jian ao cheng kuai.*)
If heat evils boil and stew the blood, static blood will congeal into lumps forming masses within the body.

Depression leads to qi stagnation. (郁则气滞。 *Yu ze qi zhi.*)
This statement can be understood in either of two ways. First, any of the four materials or yin depression may lead to qi stagnation. This is because blood stasis, dampness, phlegm, and stagnant food can all hinder and obstruct the free flow of the qi. Secondly, liver depression results in qi stagnation because the liver governs coursing and discharge. If the liver is depressed and loses control over coursing and discharge, the qi becomes stagnant.

Qi damage [causes] pain; form damage [causes] swelling. (气伤痛，形伤肿. *Qi shang tong, xing shang zhong.*)
This statement appears to be talking about traumatic injury. According to this saying, damage of the qi causes loss of free flow and, therefore, pain. However, damage of the body, as opposed to the qi, causes disruption in the free flow of water fluids and, therefore, swelling. The clinical implication of this statement seems to be that damage of the qi is less serious and damage of the form is more serious, since it typically takes a more serious injury to cause swelling as opposed to simply pain.

Qi vacuity easily lodges dampness, [while] damp depression easily brews heat. [If] dampness [and] heat lodge [and become] attached, [they] often consume [and] damage the righteous qi. (气虚易留湿，湿郁易蕴热，湿热留恋，每每耗伤正气。 *Qi xu yi liu shi, shi yu yi yun re, shi re liu lian, mei mei hao shang zheng qi.*)
Qi vacuity may lead to dampness if vacuous qi fails to move and transform water fluids. However, if dampness then inhibits the free flow of qi, this can give rise to depressive or transformative heat. This statement then goes on to say that such damp heat may consume and damage the righteous qi.

Lack of luxuriance [or construction] leads to pain. (不荣则痛。
Bu rong ze tong.)

> According to this statement, lack of constructive qi fails to nourish
> the channels and vessels properly. The channels and vessels thus
> lose their free flow, and pain is the result.

[If] the qi ascends [and] does not descend, the head [is] painful
[and] the vertex [is] diseased. (气上不下，头痛巅疾。*Qi shang
bu xia, tou tong dian ji.*)

> This statement explains that upwardly counterflowing qi accum-
> ulating in the boney box of the cranium can lead to headache. In
> fact, this is commonly a mechanism of headache in clinical practice
> where the upwardly counterflowing qi is mostly coming from the
> liver.

Hundreds of diseases are engendered from the qi. (百病皆生于
气也。*Bai bing jie sheng yu qi ye.*)

> This means that many, many diseases involve some sort of qi
> disease. In Chinese medicine, there are two basic kinds of qi disease.
> They are qi vacuity and qi stagnation, with qi counterflow being a
> further evolution of qi stagnation. In clinical practice, it is rare to find
> a patient without either of these two kinds of qi disease.

[If] the low back [and] kidneys are chilled, [they] are not able to
steam upward. [Thus,] the grain qi descends to the bottom to
become urine. (腰肾即冷，则不能蒸于上，谷气尽下为小
便。*Yao shen ji leng, ze bu neng zheng yu shang, gu qi jin xia
wei xiao bian.*)

> Kidney yang warms and steams the spleen, enabling the spleen qi to
> move and transform the finest essence of food and drink. Therefore,
> if kidney yang is vacuous, the spleen is not warmed and steamed
> properly and, hence, cannot separate clear from turbid. Instead, the
> clear descends to the lower burner with the turbid and is excreted
> as urine.

Qi vacuity leads to beating [and] stirring lacking strength; blood
depletion leads to the vessels [and] passageways not being full.
(气虚则鼓动无力，血亏则脉道不充。*Qi xu ze gu dong wu li,
xue kui ze mai dao bu chong.*)

The qi is what moves blood and fluids. Therefore, qi vacuity results in lack of strength to move these yin substances. Blood, on the other hand, nourishes the channels and vessels. Therefore, its vacuity also leads to the loss of function of the channels and vessels. Therefore, either qi or blood vacuity can lead to lack of free flow of the channels and vessels.

[If] the qi above is insufficient, the brain [will] not be full, the ears [will] be bitter [or suffer from] ringing, the head [will] be bitter from leaning, [and] the eyes [will be] dizzy. (上气不足，脑为之不满，耳为之苦鸣，头为之苦倾，目为之眩。*Shang qi bu zu, nao wei zhi by man, er wei zhi ku ming, tou wei zhi ku qing, mu wei zhi xuan.*)

For the brain to function properly, the clear qi must ascend to the brain to empower it. If the clear qi does not sufficiently ascend to fill and empower the function of the brain, then there will be problems with thinking and consciousness, the ears will hurt, the head may ache, and the eyes may not see properly. In fact, there may be vertigo.

Debility of yang qi below leads to cold reversal. (阳气衰于下则为寒厥 *Yang qi shuai yu xia ze wei han jue.*)

In this statement, cold reversal probably refers to cold shock. In other words, there is decreased or loss of consciousness with symptoms of pale face and chilled limbs. According to this statement, this is due to yang qi not residing in the lower burner correctly. This surmise is based on the fact that moxibustion on lower burner points is commonly used to treat cold shock.

Debility of yin qi below leads to heat reversal. (阴气衰于下则为热厥 *Yin qi shuai yu xia ze wei re jue.*)

If the previous statement has to do with cold shock, then this one has to do with hot shock. In this case, there is mental confusion, a red face, and hot extremities. According to this statement, hot shock has to do with insufficient yin qi in the lower burner. In clinical practice, hot shock is often treated with moxibustion at *Yong Quan* (Ki 1) in order to lead yang back down to its lower source and, thereby, once more becoming integrated and held in place by yin.

[If] visceral qi [is] insufficient, disease is in the viscera. [If] the bowel qi [is] insufficient, disease is in the bowels. [If] the channels [and] vessels [are] insufficient, disease is in the channels [and] vessels. (脏气不足，病在脏；腑气不足，病在腑；经脉不足，病在经脉。*Zang qi bu zu, bing zai zang; fu qi bu zu, bing zai fu; jing mai bu zu, bing zai jing mai.*)

> According to this statement, qi vacuity in any viscera or bowel, channel or network vessel will display signs and symptoms of that vacuity in that entity.

Qi follows fluid desertion. (气随津脱。*Qi sui jin tuo.*)

> This statement says that, if fluids desert, qi will follow these fluids and this will also lead to qi desertion. Fluid desertion refers to massive, sudden loss of fluids, such as through vomiting or diarrhea.

Viscera & Bowel Disease Mechanisms
(脏腑病机, *zang fu bing ji*)

Viscus may transmit [and] change to viscus. (脏与脏传变。*Zang yu zang zhuan bian.*)

> This means that disease may be transmitted from one viscus to another, such as spleen vacuity eventually leading to lung vacuity or liver heat eventually floating upward to accumulate in the lungs.

Viscus may transmit [and] change to bowel. (脏与腑传变。*Zang yu fu zhuan bian.*)

> This means that disease may be transmitted from viscus to bowel and vice versa. For instance heart fire may be transmitted to the small intestine and bladder, or stomach heat may be transmitted to the lungs.

Bowel may transmit [and] change to bowel. (腑与腑传变。*Fu yu fu zhuan bian.*)

> This means that disease may transmit from one bowel to another, such as from stomach to large intestine or small intestine to bladder.

Visceral disease [is] mostly vacuity. (脏病多虚。*Zang bing duo xu.*)

According to this statement, diseases of the viscera are associated more commonly with vacuity than repletion. This is especially so with the spleen and kidneys.

Bowel disease [is] mostly repletion. (腑病多实。 *Fu bing duo shi.*)
> According to this statement, most bowel diseases are due to some repletion of evil qi. Usually, this repletion is heat.

[If there is] bowel disease, the upper back will be distended. (腑病为背胀 *Fu bing wei bei zhang.*)
> This statement says that one symptom of bowel disease is distention of the upper back. In all probability, this statement is referring to the gallbladder. Cholecystitis often does refer pain to the upper back.

[If there is] visceral disease, the abdomen will be full. (脏病为腹满 *Zang bing wei fu man.*)
> Conversely, if there is a disease of the viscera, it is the abdomen which will commonly feel full.

Liver-Gallbladder Disease Mechanisms
(肝胆病机, *gan dan bing ji*)

While the liver and gallbladder may contract external damp heat, the overwhelming majority of internally engendered liver-gallbladder pathologies stem from liver depression. Liver depression refers to qi stagnation within the liver. Thus the liver loses its control over coursing and discharge.

Liver depression may transform into fire. (肝郁化火 *Gan yu hua huo.*)
> Liver depression is an abbreviation of liver depression qi stagnation and qi is inherently warm. If the liver becomes depressed and the qi stagnant, the qi accumulates in the body. When enough of this qi accumulates in one place, the person experiences the heat of this stagnant qi. This is called depressive heat or depressive fire depending on how hot the heat evils are, fire being hotter and more virulent than heat.

Liver yang may transform into wind. (肝阳化风 *Gan yang hua feng.*)

> This means that ascendant liver yang hyperactivity (肝阳上亢, *gan yang shang kang*) may transform into internal stirring of liver wind (肝风内动, *gan feng nei dong*).

Liver yang may transform into fire. (肝阳化火 *Gan yang hua huo.*)

Ascendant liver yang hyperactivity may also transform into liver fire flaming upward (肝阳上亢也化肝火上炎, *Gan yang shang kang ye hua gan huo shang yan.*)

Liver vacuity leads to blood disease. (肝虚则血病 *Gan xu ze xue bing.*)

> Liver vacuity means liver yin-blood vacuity. If there is liver blood vacuity, then, ipso facto, the blood is diseased.

Liver vacuity leads to head dizziness. (肝虚则头眩 *Gan xu ze tou xuan.*)

> As stated above, liver vacuity is liver yin-blood vacuity. If liver yin or blood are incapable of controlling yang, yang hyperactivity may give rise to the engenderment of wind resulting in dizziness.

Liver disease spreads to the spleen. (肝病传脾 *Gan bing chuan pi.*)

Liver depression leads to spleen vacuity, [and] spleen vacuity leads to loss of normalcy of movement [and] transformation. (肝郁则脾虚，脾虚则运化失常。 *Gan yu ze pi xu, pi xu ze yun hua shi chang.*)

> This statement is an extension of the preceding one. When the liver becomes depressed, it is typically the spleen and/or stomach which are next affected.

[If one] sees disease of the liver, know [that] the liver transmits to the spleen. [Therefore, one] must first replete the spleen. (见肝之病，知肝传脾，当先实脾。 *Jian gan zhi bing, zhi gan zhuan pi, dang xian shi pi.*)

This statement from the *Nei Jing* (*Inner Classic*) is the classic saying indicating that liver depression typically causes spleen vacuity.

Liver disease is spleen disease. (肝病为脾病 *Gan bing wei pi bing.*)

This statement is even more succinct. If there is liver disease, there will be spleen disease.

Liver wood may attack the stomach. (肝木犯胃 *Gan mu fan wei.*)

Liver qi may invade the stomach. (肝气犯胃 *Gan qi fan wei.*)

If liver depression qi stagnation counterflows horizontally, it may assail or invade the stomach causing the stomach to counterflow upward and/or become hot.

Liver qi counterflowing upward [and] clashing with the stomach makes for vomiting. (肝气上逆，冲胃为呕。 *Gan qi shang ni, chong wei wei ou.*)

When the liver counterflows horizontally and assails the stomach, nausea and vomiting commonly occur.

Liver fire may invade the stomach. (肝火犯胃 *Gan huo fan wei.*)

This saying may be explained in the same two ways. Either liver fire travels over the control cycle to assail the stomach or liver fire floats upward to accumulate in the stomach. In the second case, the liver is considered to reside below the stomach, even in the lower burner.

Liver fire may invade the lungs. (肝火犯肺 *Gan huo fan fei.*)

Based on the control cycle, liver fire may rebel against the control of the lungs, thus invading or assailing the lungs. This saying may also be simply explained by liver fire floating upward anatomically to assail the lungs.

Liver qi flowing freely leads to the heart qi [being] harmonious, [while] liver qi stagnation leads to a lack of heart qi. (肝气通则心气和，肝气滞则心气乏。 *Gan qi tong ze xin qi he, gan qi zhi ze xin qi fa.*)

This statement explains how liver depression can lead to heart qi vacuity. In fact, liver depression causing heart qi vacuity usually acts via the spleen. In this case, liver depression causes spleen qi vacuity which then causes heart qi vacuity.

Liver fire effulgence leads to excessive coursing and discharge. (肝火旺则疏泄太过 *Gan huo wang ze shu xie tai guo*.)

Liver fire effulgence typically evolves from liver depression transforming heat. However, once there is fire in the liver, the liver becomes hyperactive and, therefore, overcourses and overdischarges. For instance, according to Qin Bo-wei, fulminant anger, a common symptom of liver fire, is a symptom of the liver's overcoursing and overdischarging.

Liver yin insufficiency leads to liver yang effulgence and exuberance. (肝阴不足则肝阳旺盛 *Gan yin bu zu ze gan yang wang sheng*.)

This is basic yin-yang theory. If liver yin fails to control liver yang, liver yang will become effulgent and exuberant.

[If] earth is damp and wood is depressed, the liver will not orderly reach. (土湿木郁，木不条达 *Tu shi mu yu, mu bu tiao da*.)

If earth is damp, this means that the spleen is damp or that spleen dysfunction has engendered dampness. In any case, this dampness will hinder and obstruct the free flow of the qi. Further, if liver qi is depressed because of unfulfilled desires, lack of nourishment by blood, or any other cause, the qi will also become stagnant. Thus, when both dampness and liver depression qi stagnation combine, this will most definitely impede the liver's orderly reaching or spreading of the qi throughout the body.

[If] the liver loses coursing and discharge [and] the qi becomes stagnant and does not flow freely, lack of free flow leads to pain. (肝失疏泄，气滞不通，不通则痛 *Gan shi shu xie, qi zhi bu tong, bu tong ze tong*.)

According to this statement, liver depression leads to qi stagnation and qi stagnation is, ipso facto, a lack of free flow of the qi. Hence, liver depression qi stagnation may and often does lead to pain.

Liver heat leads to red eyes; little heat leads to itching; serious heat leads to pain. (肝热则目赤，热微则痒，热甚则痛 *Gan re ze mu chi, re wei ze yang, re shen ze tong.*)
  Because heat naturally has a tendency to float or ascend in the body, liver heat may follow the liver channel and ascend to the eyes, making the eyes red. Further, according to this statement, minor liver heat leads to itching of the skin, while severe liver heat leads to pain. In the latter case, severe liver heat depressed within the skin and flesh causes lack of free flow of the local qi and blood, thus resulting in pain.

Lower burner disease necessarily shifts to [or pushes onto] the liver and kidneys. (下焦者病须推肝肾 *Xia jiao zhe bing xu tui gan shen.*)
  The liver and kidneys are the main organs located within the lower burner. According to this statement, diseases in the uterus, intestines, and bladder may eventually affect the liver and/or kidneys. For instance, damp heat in the uterus may eventually affect the liver and/or kidneys.

[If there is] liver depression and rib-side pain, the liver network vessels within have static blood. (肝郁胁痛乃肝络中有淤血 *Gan yu xie tong nai gan luo zhong you yu xue.*)
  The intercostal spaces are traversed by the liver network vessels. Therefore, if there is liver depression qi stagnation with rib-side pain, there may be static blood within the liver network vessels.

Upward counterflow of the liver qi leads all the qi to counterflow. (肝气上逆则诸气皆逆 *Gan qi shang ni ze zhu qi jie ni.*)
  Upward counterflow of the liver qi can cause upward counterflow of the stomach and/or lungs as well. In addition, upward counterflow of the liver qi may also lead to stirring and upward counterflow of life-gate/ministerial fire.

Liver qi depression and blood stagnation turn into stasis. (肝气郁而血滞成淤 *Gan qi yu er xue zhi cheng yu.*)
  If the liver is depressed, then the qi is stagnant. Because the qi moves the blood, qi stagnation may eventually lead to blood stasis.

Drum distention is caused by angry qi damaging the liver. (鼓胀
由于怒气伤肝。 *Gu zhang you yu nu qi shang gan.*)
Drum distention is an especially severe form of abdominal
distention. According to this statement, it is caused by anger leading
to liver depression qi stagnation.

Liver vacuity engenders cold. (肝虚生寒 *Gan xu sheng han.*)
Whether there is a liver qi or yang vacuity pattern is highly debated
within the Chinese medical literature. If the liver channel contracts
cold, it causes mounting (疝, *shan*) conditions. However, most
Chinese authorities explain this as a combination of liver depression
qi stagnation with vacuity cold due to a spleen-kidney dual vacuity
rather than a true liver vacuity *per se.*

[If] the liver loses its orderly reaching [and] depression affects
the root channels, this leads to the appearance of rib-side pain
and breast distention. (肝失条达，郁于本经则见胁痛乳胀
Gan shi tiao da, yu yu ben jing ze jian xie tong ru zhang.)
Basically, there is no rib-side pain or breast distention without liver
depression qi stagnation. As such, these are extremely important
and reliable symptoms of liver depression.

Liver qi vacuity leads to fear. (肝气虚则恐。 *Gan qi xu ze kong.*)

Liver vacuity leads to gallbladder timidity. (肝虚则胆怯 *Gan xu
ze dan qie.*)
Again, it is questionable whether there is any liver qi or yang vacuity
pattern. A more probable explanation of this statement is that liver
depression and its attendant spleen vacuity results in a heart qi and
blood vacuity and, therefore, a lack of courage. *Ergo*, there is
timidity. In this case, the concept of gallbladder timidity is based on
the ancient relationship between the gall and bravery. However,
now, this concept is simply used as a shorthand for the preceding
more complex disease mechanism resulting in a lack of heart spirit
and, therefore, courage.

Liver and kidney vacuity [and] damp heat stopping up the lower
burner cause lack of strength in the feet and knees. (肝肾虚，湿
热壅于下焦，故脚膝无力 *Gan shen xu, shi re yong yu xia jiao,
gu jiao xi wu li.*)

The combination of liver-kidney dual vacuity with damp heat pouring downward is a commonly seen complicated pattern in a number of wilting conditions, such as rheumatoid arthritis and multiple sclerosis.

[If] liver depression upbears fire, [there may be] afternoon tidal heat. (肝郁升火，午后潮热 *Gan yu sheng huo, wu hou chao re.*)
According to this statement, liver depression transforming fire is a potential cause of afternoon tidal heat. However, afternoon tidal heat is usually associated with yin vacuity, in which case fire has damaged yin.

Liver heat leads to gallbladder discharge [and] bitter mouth. (肝热则胆泄口苦 *Gan re ze dan xie kou ku.*)
The liver and gallbladder are mutually related, the gallbladder qi is dependent on the liver qi, and the gallbladder's function is to store the gall or bile. If the liver is hot, then it and the gallbladder tend to be hyperactive. In that case, the gallbladder oversecretes bile and this results in a bitter taste in the mouth. In fact, this is a very reliable symptom in clinical practice. Liver-gallbladder heat is the only cause of a specifically bitter taste in the mouth.

[When] apt to vomiting, [if] the vomitus has a bitter [taste]… evils are in the gallbladder [and] counterflow is in the stomach. Discharge of bile leads to a bitter [taste in] the mouth. Stomach qi counterflow leads to bitter vomit. (善呕，呕有苦… 邪在胆，逆在胃，胆液泄则口苦，胃气逆则呕苦。 *Shan ou, ou you ku… xie zai dan, ni zai wei, dan ye xie ze kou ku, wei qi ni ze ou ku.*)
As seen above, liver assailing the stomach often leads to nausea and vomiting, while liver heat shifted to the gallblabber leads to a bitter taste. Therefore, bitter tasting vomiting is due to liver heat or fire attacking the stomach.

Liver fire overwhelming the lungs leads to cough. (肝火乘肺则咳 *Gan huo cheng fei ze ke.*)
If liver fire counterflows upward, it assails the lungs causing the lungs to lose their depurative downbearing. Instead the lung qi also counterflows upward and coughing occurs.

Liver blood vacuity leads to steaming bones and tidal heat. (肝血虚则骨蒸潮热 *Gan xue xu ze gu zheng chao re.*)

> Steaming bones and tidal heat are both yin vacuity symptoms. Here, we need to remember that the blood and essence share a common source and the liver and kidneys share a common source, and that kidney yin vacuity in clinical practice is actually liver blood-kidney yin vacuity. Thus liver blood vacuity leads to steaming bones and tidal fever.

[If] the liver and kidney network vessels are vacuous, low back pain will not stop. (肝肾络虚腰痛不止 *Gan shen luo xu yao tong bu zhi.*)

> The low back is the mansion of the kidneys, and the liver and kidneys share a common source. Therefore, if the liver and kidney network vessels are vacuous, low back pain may be a result.

Heart-Small Intestine Disease Mechanisms
(心小肠病机, *xin xiao chang bing ji*)

Heart blood insufficiency leads to heart fire effulgence [and] exuberance. (心血不足则心火旺盛 *Xin xue bu zu ze xin huo wang sheng.*)

> In this statement, the word "blood" stands not just for blood but also yin. Since yin controls yang, if heart yin-blood is vacuous and insufficient, heart yang may become hyperactive and even transform into fire. Thus there is heart fire effulgence.

Heart fire upbearing upward causes sores to arise in the mouth [and] tongue. (心火上升，故口舌生疮 *Xin huo shang sheng, gu kou she sheng chuang.*)

> The tongue is the sprout of the heart and, in particular, the tip of the tongue corresponds to the heart. Therefore, red, inflamed sores on the tip of the tongue are a common and reliable sign of heart fire flaming upward.

Blood not nourishing the heart leads to heart palpitations [and] little sleep. (血不养心则心悸少寐 *Xue bu yang xin ze xin ji shao mei.*)

As seen above, the heart spirit is nothing other than an accumu-lation of heart qi and the heart qi governs the stirring or beating of the heart and its vessels. If blood fails to nourish the heart qi, then the heart spirit will become disquieted, resulting in insomnia, and the heart qi will not stir properly, resulting in palpitations.

[If] the construction [and] blood are consumed internally, [they will] not nourish the heart. (营血内耗无以养心 *Ying xue nei hao wu yi yang xin.*)

The heart qi is constructed and nourished by the constructive qi and the blood. Therefore, if the heart does not obtain sufficient constructive qi and blood, it will be malnourished and so will not function correctly.

Heart-kidney vacuity detriment [results in] vacuity wind internally stirring. (心肾亏损， 虚风内动 *Xin shen kui sun, xu feng nei dong.*)

Heart-kidney vacuity detriment most commonly refers to heart-kidney yin vacuity. If yin fails to control yang, the yang qi may stir frenetically, thus engendering internal wind.

Heart fire exuberance leads to the spirit not being quiet. (心火盛则神不安 *Xin huo sheng ze shen bu an.*)

Spirit is qi and, therefore, naturally moves. However, it should not move either too much or too little. Fire, an extreme form of heat, causes the qi to move frenetically. Therefore, the spirit is not quiet.

Heart qi vacuity leads to the spirit not keeping its abode. (心气虚则神无所依 *Xin qi xu ze shen wu suo yi.*)

If the heart qi does not construct the heart spirit, it has nowhere to gather and accumulate. Thus it fails to keep its abode.

Heart qi vacuity leads to sorrow; repletion leads to smiling and laughing without stop. (心气虚则悲，实则笑不休 *Xin qi xu ze bei, shi ze xiao bu xiu.*)

According to this statement, lack of heart qi or leads to sorrow, while abundant heart qi or spirit leads to happiness. Here repletion is used in a good, healthy sense.

[If] evils [cause] chaos of the spirit brightness [*i.e.*, consciousness, and] angry qi surges [and] stirs, there will be raving, cursing and calumny. (邪乱神明，怒气冲动，妄言骂詈. *Xie luan shen ming, nu qi chong dong, wang yan ma zi.*)

According to this statement, if evil qi causes the heart qi to move chaotically, and angry qi, *i.e.*, liver qi or liver fire, cause the heart spirit to stir frenetically, then there will be raving, cursing, and the shouting of abuse. In this case, evil qi most probably refers to phlegm obstructing the heart.

Heart heat [causes] the red color and spillage of the network vessels. (心热者色赤而络脉溢 *Xin re zhe se chi er luo mai yi.*)

Spillage of the network vessels refers to pathological bleeding, while the red color means a red facial complexion or red skin lesions. In this case, because the heart governs the blood, heat in the heart has entered the blood aspect, making the blood move frenetically. This has damaged the network vessels and also caused the blood to move to the exterior.

Heart fire exuberance [causes] vacuity vexation and no sleep. (心火盛者虚烦而不寐 *Xin huo sheng zhe xu fan er bu mei.*)

If heat or fire evils accumulate within the heart and damage and consume heart yin, they will also cause the spirit to stir frenetically and be disquieted. Therefore, there is vexation and insomnia.

Vexation pertains to the heart; agitation pertains to the kidneys. (烦属于心，躁属于肾 *Fan shu yu xin, zao shu yu shen.*)

Vexation is a subjective feeling or symptom of a dry, irritating or vexing heat in the center of the chest. Agitation is an objective sign. It refers to fidgeting or moving restlessly. According to this statement, vexation pertains to the heart, or more specifically, heat within the heart, while agitation pertains to the kidneys, kidney yin vacuity failing to control the stirring of yang.

All painful [and] itching sores pertain to the heart. (诸痛痒疮，皆属于心 *Zhu tong yang chuang, jie shu yu xin.*)

According to this statement from the *Nei Jing (Inner Classic)*, because the heart governs the blood and most sores are due to heat in the blood, it is said that all painful, itching sores pertain to the heart. In contemporary clinical practice, this statement must be taken with a grain of salt.

Heart vacuity leads to a fine pulse. (心虚则脉细 *Xin xu ze mai xi.*)

> A fine pulse is primarily an indicator that the substantial contents of the vessels, the yin blood and fluids, are insufficient, and the heart governs the blood. Therefore, a heart yin-blood vacuity leads to a fine pulse.

The heart may shift heat to the small intestine. (心移热于小肠 *Xin yi re yu xiao chang.*)

> The heart and small intestine are mutually related. One is yin and the other is yang. Because heat is a yang evil, it has no inherent affinity for the yin heart. Therefore, heat may be transmitted from the heart to the yang small intestine with which heat does have more of an intrinsic affinity.

[If] cold qi lodges in the small intestine, the small intestine [will] not obtain production [and] gathering. Therefore, [there will be] abdominal pain. (寒气客小肠，小肠不得成聚，故后腹痛矣。 *Han qi ke xiao chang, xiao chang bu de cheng ju, gu hou fu tong yi.*)

> According to this statement, cold lodged in the small intestine will cause abdominal pain. The statement that the small intestine does not obtain production and gathering seems to indicate that this cold is vacuity cold.

[If] cold qi lodges between the intestines [and] stomach [or] below the membrane origin, the blood [will] not obtain scattering [and] the small network vessels [will become] tense [and] drawn, thus resulting [in] pain. (寒气客于肠胃之间，膜原之下，血不得散，小络急引，故痛。 *Han qi ke yu chang wei zhi jian, mo yuan zhi xia, xue bu de san, xiao luo ji yin, gu tong.*)

> Because cold is constricting and tension-causing in nature, cold causes the blood flow to lose its free flow. If there is cold lodged in the abdomen, then there may be abdominal pain.

Spleen-Stomach Disease Mechanisms
(脾胃病机, *pi wei bing ji*)

Stomach vacuity leads to the five viscera, six bowels, 12 channels, 15 network vessels, and the four limbs all not obtaining the construction [and] movement of qi and the engenderment of hundreds of diseases. (胃虚则五脏，六腑，十二经，十五络，四肢皆不得营运之气，而百病生焉。*Wei xu ze wu zang, liu fu, shi er jing, shi wu luo, si zhi jie bu de ying yun zhi qi, er bai bing sheng yan.*)

In modern Chinese medicine, there is no professionally recognized pattern of stomach qi vacuity. Therefore, what this statement is really referring to is spleen-stomach qi vacuity. Because the spleen and stomach are the latter heaven source of the engenderment and transformation of all the qi and blood in the body, their vacuity may lead to the nonconstruction and malnourishment of any organ, tissue, or vessel in the body and hence the causation of all sorts of diseases.

Stomach heat leads to the dispersion of grains [and] a predilection for hunger. (胃热则消谷善饥。*Wei re ze xiao gu shan ji.*)

This statement means that stomach heat leads to a rapid dispersion of food and drink and, therefore, a tendency to rapid hunger and a large appetite.

Stomach heat may exploit the heart. (胃热乘心 *Wei re cheng xin.*)

Because all heat floats upward in the body, stomach heat may ascend to accumulate in and harass the heart. This is a commonly seen occurrence in clinical practice, especially in men.

Spleen vacuity leads to loose stools. (脾虚则便溏 *Pi xu ze bian tang.*)

Spleen qi not upbearing leads to diarrhea. (脾气不升则泻 *Pi qi bu sheng ze xie.*)

If the spleen qi is vacuous and weak, it will not upbear the finest essence engendered and transformed from food and drink. Instead, the clear may descend with the turbid, causing loose stools or diarrhea. In clinical practice, spleen qi vacuity is a commonly seen cause of loose stools and chronic diarrhea.

[If] there is central qi vacuity cold, taking chilled [foods and drinks] leads to diarrhea. (中气虚寒，得冷则泻 *Zhong qi xu han, de leng ze xie.*)

> If the spleen and stomach qi are already suffering from vacuity cold, taking chilled foods may aggravate this situation even more and lead to diarrhea where previously there was none.

Stomach qi counterflowing upward leads to vomiting. (胃气上逆则吐 *Wei qi shang ni ze tu.*)

> In Chinese medicine, vomiting is nothing other than the outward manifestation of the upward counterflow of the stomach qi which ordinarily should downbear and descend.

[If] the spleen is constantly insufficient, the kidneys will be constantly vacuous. (脾常不足肾常虚 *Pi chang bu zu shen chang xu.*)

> Because former and latter heavens are mutually rooted, spleen vacuity over time may evolve into a spleen-kidney dual vacuity. In this case, the spleen qi and kidney yang are both vacuous.

Spleen disease leads to downward flow [of dampness] over-whelming the kidneys. (脾病则下流乘肾 *Pi bing ze xia liu cheng shen.*)

> Spleen disease here refers to spleen qi vacuity with internal engenderment of damp evils. Since damp evils tend to descend, they seep downward from the middle to the lower burner where they may overwhelm the kidneys. In this case, there is polyuria which may eventually lead to kidney qi and/or yang vacuity.

Stomach cold leads to food not moving. (胃寒则食不运 *Wei han ze shi bu yun.*)

> If the stomach contracts cold, it will fail to move the food. Instead, the food will become stagnant within the stomach.

Middle burner harmony leads to normally flowing qi above [and] below. (中焦和则上下气顺 *Zhong jiao he ze shang xia qi shun.*)

Middle burner function is nothing other than the harmonious functioning of the spleen and stomach. The spleen qi should upbear and
the stomach qi should downbear. Thus, the qi flows normally up
and down or above and below.

Spleen vacuity leads to no taste for grains [and] food. (脾虚则谷食无味 *Pi xu ze gu shi wu wei.*)

The spleen connects with the mouth and tongue and the sense of
taste corresponds to the spleen. Therefore, if the spleen is vacuous
there is a lack of taste or a bland taste within the mouth. In clinical
practice, lack of taste is a fairly reliable symptom of spleen vacuity
when it occurs. However, there is often spleen vacuity with no
change in one's ability to taste.

Spleen vacuity engenders dampness; stomach weakness engenders phlegm. (脾虚生湿，胃弱生痰 *Pi xu sheng shi, wei ruo sheng tan.*)

Spleen qi vacuity failing to move and transform water fluids results
in the collecting of dampness. Then why does this statement go on
to say that stomach weakness engenders phlegm as if the spleen
plays no part in this process? This is because the stomach qi downbears turbidity, and phlegm is an even more turbid form of dampness. In actuality, the second part of this saying plays no part in
clinical practice.

Vomiting damages the stomach; diarrhea damages the spleen. (呕吐伤胃，泄泻伤脾 *Ou tu shang wei, xie xie shang pi.*)

Enduring vomiting damages stomach yin and the stomach is averse
to dryness. Enduring diarrhea damages the spleen qi.

Spleen vacuity engenders phlegm, stomach dryness engenders fire. (脾虚生痰，胃燥生火 *Pi xu sheng tan, wei zao sheng huo.*)

Above we have seen how spleen vacuity may engender phlegm.
The second part of this saying goes on to state that stomach
dryness engenders fire. In fact, in clinical practice, it is common to
see a vacuous and damp spleen along with a hot, dry stomach.

[If] the spleen and stomach have heat, this leads to mouth odor.(脾胃有热则口臭 *Pi wei you re ze kou chou.*)

Heat in the spleen and stomach causes more rottening and ripening of the food in the stomach and thus bad breath. In general, bad
breath is a reliable sign of stomach heat.

Repletion leads to *yang ming* [disease], while vacuity leads to *tai
yin*. (实则阳明，虚则太阴 *Shi ze yang ming, xu ze tai yin*.)
This saying implies that the stomach is most likely to suffer from
repletions, such as food stagnation and heat, while the spleen is
most likely to suffer from qi vacuity.

Free flowing intestines lead to stomach harmony [and] stomach
harmony leads to phlegm dampness being downborne below.
(肠通则胃和，胃和则痰湿下降 *Chang tong ze wei he, wei he
ze tan shi xia jiang*.)
The stomach and intestines are closely connected. According to this
statement, if the intestines are not freely flowing, as when there is
constipation, this can adversely affect the stomach. In real life,
constipation is often associated with stomach heat. However, if the
stomach qi is harmonious or downbearing, then turbidity is normally
downborne, and phlegm dampness is species of turbidity.

Lack of stomach harmony leads to lying down [or sleep] not
being quiet. (胃不和则卧不安 *Wei bu he ze qo bu an*.)
If food becomes stagnant in the stomach, this stagnant food may
hinder the inward and downward movement of the defensive qi at
night. Because the defensive qi is part of the global yang qi of the
body, yang qi is not embraced and smothered by yin internally. This
then leads to insomnia.

Penetrating qi spontaneously below assailing the stomach leads
to hiccup. (冲气自下犯胃则呃 *Chong qi zi xia fan wei ze e*.)
The penetrating qi in this statement refers to the qi of the chong
mai, and the chong mai and stomach channels meet in the lower
burner at *Qi Jie* (St 30). If the penetrating qi surges into the
stomach channel, it may cause upward counterflow of the stomach
qi, thus resulting in hiccups.

[If] the middle burner's upbearing [and] downbearing is not
uninhibited, the lower burner's conveyance [and] conduction
will suffer obstruction. (中焦升降不利，下焦传导受阻 *Zhong
jiao sheng jiang bu li, xia jiao chuan dao shou zu*.)

According to this statement, if the spleen and stomach's upbearing and downbearing are not freely flowing, this will cause obstruction to the conveyance and conduction of the large intestine. The result of this obstruction is constipation.

Spleen vacuity leads to no movement; kidney vacuity leads to no treasuring. (脾虚则不运，肾虚则不藏 *Pi xu ze bu yun, shen xu ze bu cang.*)

According to this statement, spleen vacuity leads to nonmovement of the finest essence of food and drink or water fluids. Kidney vacuity leads to nontreasuring of the essence. The yin-yang dichotomy that is implied by this saying is that movement is opposed to treasuring which is a species of nonmovement.

The root of diarrhea is nothing other than in the spleen [and] stomach. (泄泻之本，无不由于脾胃。 *Xie xie zhi ben, wu bu you yu pi wei.*)

This saying emphasizes that the root of diarrhea is spleen-stomach dysfunction even though diarrhea itself exits from the large intestine.

Stomach vessel repletion leads to distention; vacuity leads to diarrhea. (胃脉实则胀，虚则泄。 *Wei mai shi ze zhang, xu ze xie.*)

If the stomach (channel) is replete, there will be abdominal distention. However, if the stomach channel is vacuous, there will be diarrhea.

[If] the tai yin spleen channel contracts dampness, water [will be] discharged [and] pour downwards, the body [will be] slightly heavy [and] slightly full, [and] thus [there is] weakness, and lack of strength, no desire to drink or eat, sudden diarrhea without number, and nontransformation of water and grain. (太阴脾经受湿，水泄注下，体微重微满，因弱无力，不欲饮食，暴泄无数，水谷不化。 *Tai yin pi jing shou shi, shui xie zhu xia, ti wei zhong wei man, yin ruo wu li, bu yu yin shi, bao xie wu shu, shui gu bu hua.*)

According to this statement, if the spleen (channel) contracts damp evils, this dampness will descend to the lower half of the body resulting in heaviness, fullness, weakness and lack of strength, lack of appetite, sudden diarrhea, and undigested food in the stools.

Even though these last two statements seem to be speaking about the spleen and stomach channels as opposed to the spleen and stomach organs, the symptomology given has to do with the organs, not their channels.

Lung-Large Intestine Disease Mechanisms
(肺大肠病机, *fei da chang bing ji*)

The lungs losing their clearing [and] depurating leads to coughing. (肺失清肃则为咳嗽 *Fei shi qing su ze wei ke sou.*)
If, for any reason, the lungs lose their clearing and depurating or depurating and downbearing, the lung qi counterflows upward causing cough.

Lung vacuity leads to coughing. (肺虚则咳嗽 *Fei xu ze ke sou.*)
Lung vacuity is one specific reason why the lungs might lose their depurating and downbearing.

Lung qi vacuity leads to nasal congestion not disinhibited. (肺气虚则鼻塞不利 *Fei qi xu ze bi sai bu li.*)
The nose is the orifice of the lungs. If the lung qi is vacuous, then it does not flow freely to the nose. Instead, the nose is congested and its flow is inhibited.

[If] the lungs lose their administrative discipline, the water pathways will not be disinhibited. (肺失治节，水道不利 *Fei shi zhu jie, shui dao bu li.*)
The downward diffusion of the lung qi keeps the water passageways freely flowing and uninhibited. Therefore, if the function of the lung qi becomes unregulated, the lungs may lose their control over the flow of the water passageways.

Lung qi vacuity leads to insecurity [or lack of consolidation] of the interstices. (肺气虚则腠理不固 *Fei qi xu ze cou li bu gu.*)
The defensive qi is emitted by and is part of the lung qi. Therefore, lung qi vacuity leads to defensive qi vacuity. Because it is the defensive qi which opens and closes the pores (气门, *qi men*) and closely packs the interstices (腠理, *cou li*), a defensive qi vacuity leads to insecurity of the interstices.

[If,] in the upper burner, the lungs lose their diffusion [and] transformation, in the lower burner, intestinal humors will then wither. (上焦肺失宣化，下焦肠液就枯 *Shang jiao fei shi xuan hua, xia jiao chang ye jiu ku.*)

> The lungs and large intestine are mutually related, yin and yang, interior and exterior. In addition, the lung qi diffuses and down-bears fluids. Therefore, if the lung qi loses its control over the downward diffusion of fluids, the large intestine will not receive its proper moistening. Hence the intestinal humors will be dry and withered and constipation will typically be the result.

[If] the lungs have hidden heat, there is frequent vomiting of blood; [if] the stomach has damp heat, there is frequent cough. (肺有伏热时常吐血，胃有湿热时常咳嗽 *Fei you fu re shi chang tu xue, wei you shi re shi chang ke sou.*)

> According to this saying, deep-lying or hidden heat in the lungs damages the network vessels of the lungs causing hemoptysis. This part of this statement is the Chinese medical explanation of hemoptysis in tuberculosis or pulmonary consumption. The second part of the saying states that stomach damp heat leads to frequent coughing. This is because heat tends to float upward to the lungs, thus disturbing the lungs' depurating and downbearing.

The lungs receiving fire damage leads to qi counterflow causing cough. (肺受火伤则气逆为咳 *Fei shou huo shang ze qi ni wei ke.*)

> This statement is similar to the second part of the preceding statement. Fire floating upwards to accumulate in the lungs or fire engendered within the lungs themselves due to depression may cause the lung qi to counterflow upward, thus resulting in cough.

Lung vacuity leads to shortness of breath, profuse phlegm, panting, and cough. (肺虚则气少，痰多，喘咳 *Fei xu ze qi shao, tan duo, chuan ke.*)

> According to this statement, lung vacuity leads to scanty qi or shortness of breath. However, because the lung qi is insufficient to diffuse and downbear water fluids, these collect and congeal into phlegm. Then, because of both a lack of qi and the presence of phlegm blocking the function of the lungs, there is panting and coughing or asthma.

Counterflow leads to damage of the lungs. (逆之则伤肺。*Ni zhi ze shang fei.*)

> Because the lung qi is supposed to downbear and descend, any upward counterflow in the body may potentially damage the lungs leading to lung qi counterflow as well.

Lung yang vacuity leads to easy catching cold. (肺阳虚，则易感冒。*Fei yang xu, ze yi gan mao.*)

> Lung yang vacuity is synonymous with a defensive qi vacuity. Thus, if the defensive qi is vacuous and the exterior is not secured, evils easily enter and the person easily contracts a cold.

Kidney-Bladder Disease Mechanisms
(肾膀胱病机, *shen pang guang bing ji*)

Kidney vacuity leads to morning diarrhea. (肾虚则晨泻 *Shen xu ze chen xie.*)

> One of the textbook signs of kidney yang vacuity is cockcrow or fifth-watch diarrhea. This refers to chronic, repeated diarrhea at daybreak. Although this is a commonly cited sign of kidney yang diarrhea, it is not commonly encountered in Western patients.

[If] kidney water is insufficient, the lungs lose their depurative downbearing. (肾水不足，肺失肃降 *Shen shui bu zu, fei shi su jiang.*)

> The kidneys are responsible for grasping or absorbing the qi downborne by the lungs. Since upbearing and downbearing are mutually reflexive, if the kidneys fail to absorb the qi sent down by the lungs, the lung qi may counterflow upward instead.

Kidney vacuity is not able to grasp [*i.e.* absorb] the qi; lung vacuity is not able to downbear the qi. (肾虚不能纳气，肺虚不能降气 *Shen xu bu neng na qi, fei xu bu neng jiang qi.*)

> In terms of respiration, as explained above, kidney vacuity may not be able to absorb the qi sent down by the lungs. However, it may also be possible that the lungs are simply too vacuous and weak to downbear the qi to the kidneys.

Kidney vacuity [results in] the penetrating qi counterflowing upward; lung vacuity [results in] phlegm heat lodging [attached to staying]. (肾虚冲气上逆，肺虚痰热留恋 *Shen xu chong qi shang ni, fei xu tan re liu lian.*)

Kidney qi vacuity leads to the chong mai or penetrating vessel qi counterflowing upward. Lung vacuity failing to clear and depurate leads to phlegm and heat lodging in the lungs.

Kidney vacuity leads to low back [and] foot soreness [and] pain. (肾虚则腰脚酸痛 *Shen xu ze yao jiao suan tong.*)

According to this statement, both low back and foot soreness and pain are symptoms of kidney vacuity. In this case, foot pain mostly refers to heel pain as in plantar fasciitis.

Essence damage leads to bone aching, wilting reversal, and the essence sometimes spontaneously precipitating. (精伤则骨酸艉厥，精时自下 *Jing shang ze gu suan wei jue, jing shi zi xia.*)

According to this statement, damage of the essence, such as by too much sex, drugs, or taxation, leads to bone pain and wilting. Wilting refers to muscular atrophy, loss of strength, and inutility. "Essence sometimes spontaneously precipitating" refers to seminal emission or seminal efflux.

Prolonged diarrhea [and] prolonged dysentery cannot but damage the kidneys. (久泄久痢无不伤肾 *Jiu xie jiu li wu bu shang shen.*)

Because it is the kidney qi which governs the closing and sealing of the rear yin or anus, enduring diarrhea or dysentery eventually wears away and consumes the kidney qi. In this case, kidney qi not securing then becomes yet another complicating mechanism of diarrhea and dysentery.

Former heaven insufficiency leads to the bones [and] marrow [being] empty [and] vacuous. (先天不足则骨髓空虚 *Xian tian bu zu ze gu sui kong xu.*)

Because the kidneys are the former heaven and the kidneys govern the bones, kidney vacuity leads to the bones and marrow being empty and vacuous.

Kidney disease [results in] large [*i.e.* upper] abdominal and small [*i.e.* lower] abdominal pain. (肾病者大腹小腹痛 *Shen bing zhe da fu xiao fu tong.*)

According to this statement, kidney disease may result in either upper or lower abdominal pain. In the case of lower abdominal pain, this is often associated with kidney yang vacuity/vacuity cold. In terms of the upper abdominal pain, the author of this statement may have been thinking of kidney stone pain.

[If] a black color appears on the face, one knows damage has reached the kidneys. (黑色现于面，则知伤及肾 *Hei se xian yu mian, ze zhi shang ji shen.*)

Both the black color and the kidneys correspond to the water element. Therefore, a black color appearing on the face may indicate a kidney vacuity.

Kidney yin vacuity leads to essence not being stored; strong liver yang leads to qi not securing [or consolidating]. (肾阴虚则精不藏，肝阳强则气不固 *Shen yin xu ze jing bu cang, gan yang qiang ze qi bu gu.*)

Kidney yin vacuity always includes within it an element of kidney qi vacuity. In addition, if there is kidney yin vacuity, yin may fail to control yang and hyperactive yang may engender heat. Therefore, essence efflux or seminal emission may be due to a combination of qi vacuity failing to secure the essence and vacuity heat forcing the fluids outside the body. Because liver yang is closely linked to life-gate/ministerial fire, this relationship is bi-directional, and flaring of life-gate/ministerial fire may lead to essence efflux, and liver yang hyperactivity may also result in seminal emission or failure to secure the essence.

The kidneys are the bar of the stomach; [if] kidney diffusion and movement is scanty, intake of food will be sluggish. (肾为胃关，肾少宣行则纳食运迟 *Shen wei wei guan, shen shao xuan xing ze na shi yun chi.*)

According to this statement, if the kidney qi does not diffuse and move water fluids properly, this will negatively affect one's appetite or intake of food.

The kidneys are the bar of the stomach; [if] the bar to this gate is not disinhibited, there will be gathering of water and other similar occurrences. (肾为胃关，关门不利姑聚水而从其类也 *Shen wei wei guan, guan men bu li gu ju shui er cong qi lei ye.*)
   Again, because the kidneys are at the end of the flow of turbid fluids originating from the stomach, if the kidney qi is not freely flowing, urination will be inhibited and water will tend to accumulate.

[If] kidney yang is devitalized, gathering water will become swelling. (肾阳不振，聚水成肿 *Shen yang bu zhen, ju shui cheng zhong.*)
   According to this statement, kidney yang vacuity will result in water collecting and causing swelling or edema.

Kidney yin vacuity [results in] the ears not hearing, the eyes not being bright, the low back and knees being aching and limp, loss of essence, [and] frenetic blood (*i.e.* bleeding). (肾阴虚者耳不聪，目不明，腰膝酸软，失精，妄血. *Shen yin xu zhe er bu cong mu bu ming, yan xi suan ruan, shi jing, wang xue.*)
   According to this statement, kidney yin vacuity can result in any of the following: deafness, loss of visual acuity, low back and knee soreness and weakness, involuntary seminal emission, or various hemorrhagic disorders.

Kidney yang vacuity [results in] yang wilting, fear of cold, water flooding, the production of phlegm, and qi panting. (肾阳虚者阳痿，畏寒，水泛为痰而气喘 *Shen yang xu zhe yang wei, wei han, shui fan wei tan er qi chuan.*)
   On the other hand, kidney yang vacuity results in impotence, fear of cold, edema, the production of phlegm, and qi panting or asthma.

Repletion leads to tai yang [disease], while vacuity leads to shao yin. (实则太阳，虚则少阴 *Shi ze tai yang, xu ze shao yin.*)
   The implication of this statement is that bladder diseases commonly are due to repletion of evils, such as damp heat, while kidney diseases are due to vacuity.

[If] the sea of marrow is insufficient, there will be dizziness of the eyes. (髓海不足，目为之眩 *Sui hai bu zu, mu wei zhi xuan.*)
According to this statement, if the kidneys are vacuous with the result that the marrow is insufficient to fill the sea of marrow or brain, there will be vertigo.

[If] the sea of marrow is insufficient, the brain spins [and] the ears ring, the shins [are] sore, [there is] dizziness, the eyes have no way to see, [and the patient is] sluggish, quiet, and sleepy. (髓海不足，则脑转耳鸣，胫酸眩冒，目无所见，懈怠安卧。 *Sui hai bu zu, ze nao zhuan er ming, jing suan xuan mao, mu wu suo jian, xie dai an wo.*)
This statement is similar to the above. However, it goes on to say that, if the sea of marrow is insufficient, there will not just be vertigo but there will also be tinnitus, sore lower extremities, dizziness, visual problems, and fatigue.

Kidney qi vacuity leads to reversal, repletion leads to distention. (肾气虚则厥，实则胀 *Shen qi xu ze jue, shi ze zhang.*)
This statement means that kidney qi (actually yang) vacuity may lead to cold spreading from the lower extremities up the body. As for kidney repletion leading to distention, in standard professional Chinese medicine, we do not believe there is any such thing as kidney repletion.

Kidney vacuity leads to urination being frequent [and] numerous. (肾虚则小便频数 *Shen xu ze xiao bian pin shu.*)
Because kidney yin and yang vacuity both include kidney qi vacuity within them, any kidney vacuity may result in urination being frequent and numerous. This is because the kidney qi does not move and transform fluids adequately. If there is kidney yin vacuity, urination may be frequent but tends to be scanty each time. If there is kidney yang vacuity, urination tends to be frequent, long, and clear.

Prolonged disease affects the kidneys. (久病及肾 *Jiu bing ji shen.*)
Any prolonged disease is bound to affect the visceral engenderment of qi and blood. Since less engenderment of the qi and blood means less latter heaven essence and more use of former heaven essence and the kidneys store the essence, any prolonged disease will eventually affect the kidneys.

[If] kidney qi does not grasp [*i.e.*, does not absorb], qi does not return to its source. (肾气不纳，气不归元 *Shen qi bu na, qi bu gui yuan.*)

> This statement has to do with the kidneys' absorption of the qi sent down by the lungs as part of the process of respiration. If the kidneys do not grasp or absorb this qi, this qi does not gather in its source, the lower burner or lower source.

Overtaxation of the sinews and bones leads to damage of the liver and kidneys. (筋骨劳则伤肝肾 *Jin gu lao ze shang gan shen.*)

> The sinews correspond to the liver and the bones correspond to the kidneys. Because this correspondence is bidirectional, overtaxation of them may lead to eventual damage of the liver and kidneys.

Kidney essence insufficiency leads to debility of the mind qi [which] is unable to communicate above with [or flow freely to] the heart, resulting in confusion, bewilderment, and aptness to forget. (肾精不足则志气衰，不能上通于心，姑迷惑善忘 *Shen jing bu zu ze zhi qi shuai, bu neng shang tong yu xin, gu mi huo shan wang.*)

> Because the end results of this disease mechanism are psychological disorders, *i.e.*, confusion, bewilderment, and forgetfulness, we have chosen to translate the seminal word 志 (*zhi*) in this instance as mind. Because the essence sent up by the kidneys to the heart helps to construct and nourish the heart spirit, insufficiency of this essence results in these mental disorders. In particular, this mechanism helps explain senile dementia or Alzheimer's disease.

The kidneys manage the two excretions; [if] the steaming and transformation of the kidneys are scanty, the two excretions will be irregular. (肾司二便，肾少蒸化则二便不调 *Shen si er bian, shen shao zheng hua ze er bian bu tiao.*)

> As we have seen above, the kidney qi helps to regulate the discharge of the feces and urine. According to this statement, if the steaming and transformation of kidney yang is less than normal, then defecation and urination will be irregular.

Kidney yang vacuity leads to steaming and transforming being inhibited. (肾阳虚则蒸化不利。 *Shen yang xu ze zheng hua bu li.*)

> Because kidney yang is the root of all yang in the body and in charge of warming and steaming all the other tissues and organs so that those tissues and organs may transform (or function), if kidney yang is vacuous, then this steaming and transforming is inhibited.

[If] kidney water is insufficient, liver wood loses [its] nourishment. (肾水不足则肝木失养。 *Shen shui bu zu ze gan mu shi yang.*)

> Because the liver and kidneys share a common source, if kidney water or yin is insufficient, then the liver will lose its enrichment and nourishment. In that case, it will not be able to carry out its yang function properly, the function of controlling coursing and discharge. Thus kidney yin vacuity is one of the disease mechanisms that can cause or aggravate liver depression qi stagnation.

Channel & Network Vessel Disease Mechanisms
(经络病机, *jing luo bing ji*)

Network vessel vacuity leads to pain. (络虚则痛 *Luo xu ze tong.*)

> Network vessel vacuity means mostly blood vacuity. If the network vessels are not adequately nourished, they cannot help move the qi and blood. If the qi and blood are not freely flowing, there is pain.

If the yang network vessels are damaged, blood will overflow outside. (阳络伤则血外溢 *Yang luo shang ze xue wai yi.*)

> In this statement, the yang network vessels imply the exterior network vessels. If these are damaged, then there is bleeding on the outside of the body.

If the yin network vessels are damaged, blood will overflow inside. (阴络伤则血内溢 *Yin luo shang ze xue nei yi.*)

> Conversely, the yin network vessels mean the network vessels in the interior of the body. If these are damaged, there will be bleeding internally.

The channels [and] vessels [can] transmit [and] change. (经脉传变。 *Jing mai chuan bian*.)

The yin [and] yang of the channels [and] vessels [may] transmit [and] change. (经脉的阴阳传变。 *Jing mai de yin yang chuan bian*.)

Similarly, disease may be transmitted and change location from one channel to another. For instance, disease in a yin channel may be transmitted to its paired yang channel and *vice versa*.

Hand [and] foot channels [and] vessels [may] transmit [and] change. (手足经脉传变。 *Shou zu jing mai chuan bian*.)

Disease can be spread and transmitted from a hand channel to its paired foot channel and *vice versa*.

Miscellaneous Disease Mechanisms
(杂感病机, *za gan bing ji*)

Disease evils [may] exit [and] enter. (病邪出入。 *Bing xie chu ru*.)

Disease evils may both enter and exit the body. However, this statement also implies that disease evils may move from exterior to interior and interior to exterior.

Exterior evils [may] enter the interior. (表邪入里。 *Biao xie ru li*.)

Exterior evils do not necessarily stay in the exterior. They may enter deeper into the body, entering the interior or the viscera and bowels.

Interior evils may exit to the exterior. (里邪出表。 *Li xie chu biao*.)

Interior evils may also, sometimes, move from interior to exterior. This is especially seen in warm diseases where there are deep-lying evils in the interior. As they become active, they may move to the exterior, resulting in skin lesions and rashes.

Disease locations [can] transmit [and] change. (病位传变。 *Bing wei chuan bian.*)

> Diseases do not always stay in the same place. For instance, a disease located in the spleen may transmit to the kidneys, thus resulting in both the spleen and kidneys being diseased. Or a disease located in the qi may transmit to the blood as in the case of qi stagnation leading to blood stasis.

The three burners [can] transmit [and] change. (三焦传变。 *San jiao chuan bian.*)

The three burners disease location [may] transmit [and] change. (三焦病位传变。 *San jiao bing wei chuan bian.*)

> These two statements mostly apply to warm disease theory. Accordingly, a warm evil may be transmitted from upper, to middle, to lower burners or the other way round. Even outside of warm disease theory, a disease which started in one burner may eventually affect other burners.

The defensive, qi, constructive, [and] blood [can] transmit [and] change. (卫气营血传变。 *Wei qi ying xue chuan bian.*)

> The defensive, qi, constructive, and blood are the four aspects of warm disease theory. According to this theory, warm evils may transmit from the defensive to the qi, from the qi to the constructive, and from the constructive to the blood as the pathogens work their way deeper and deeper into the body. However, sometimes this progression can work in the opposite direction, as with AIDS.

The form [and] viscera, internal [and] external [may] transmit [and] change. (形脏内外传变。 *Xing zang nei wai chuan bian.*)

> According to this statement, disease evils may be transmitted and change location between the body and the viscera, the internal and external.

A recent external contraction may stir a hidden [*i.e.*, deep-lying] evil. (新感引动伏邪 *Xin gan yin dong fu xie.*)

> According to this statement, a new external contraction may cause a deep-lying or hidden evil which has been relatively latent to become active. Thus the new evil may be said to have stirred up the hidden evil.

Deep-lying qi [causes] warm diseases. (伏气温病。*Fu qi wen bing.*)

Deep-lying or hidden qi tends to cause warm diseases when it erupts or becomes visible.

Deep-lying [evils] later emit. (伏而后发。*Fu er hou fa.*)

This statement means that deep-lying or hidden evils enter the body at one time but cause disease at a later time.

All diseases [are] mostly engendered by depression. (诸病多生于郁 *Zhu bing duo sheng yu yu.*)

"Depression" here may mean any of the six depressions (六郁, *liu yu*). The six depressions are qi (气, *qi*), blood (血, *xue*), dampness (湿, *shi*), phlegm (痰, *tan*), food (食, *shi*), and fire (火, *huo*). However, of the six depressions, qi depression or stagnation is the most common and can lead to or aggravate any of the other five. Therefore, it is rare to find a disease which does not include some element of depression.

Turbid evils harm the clear. (浊邪害清 *Zhuo xie hai qing.*)

Turbid evils include rheum/dampness, phlegm, and food stagnation. Since phlegm is created from dampness and the spleen is averse to dampness, rheum/dampness and phlegm can damage the spleen, thus harming the upbearing of the clear. Since food stagnation impedes the free flow of the spleen and stomach qi, it too may damage the spleen and hinder the upbearing of the clear. Thus, turbid evils harm the clear.

Repletion may transform into vacuity. (由实转虚。*You shi zhuan xu.*)

This means that a replete disease over time may transform into a vacuity disease. For instance, a lung disease may start out as a wind cold repletion. However, if the evils persist and endure, eventually, the lung qi may be damaged resulting in a lung qi vacuity cough.

Vacuity may result in repletion. (因虚致实。*Yin xu zhi shi.*)

This means that because of a vacuity, this may result in a repletion. For instance, spleen vacuity may result in the engenderment of dampness or phlegm, both repletions. Or, due to defensive vacuity, wind evils may enter and lodge in the body. These wind evils are a repletion.

Cold may transform into heat. (由寒化热。*You han hua re.*)
Because of the theory of similar transformation, cold evils lodged in the body may transform into heat because the body's host or ruling qi is warm.

Heat may transform into cold. (由热转寒。*You re zhuan han.*)
It is also possible for exuberant heat evils to so damage the righteous yang of the body that the yang qi becomes vacuous and debilitated. In that case, there will be vacuity cold.

[If] clear yang does not upbear, there will be heaviness of the head. (清阳不升，则头为之重 *Qing yang bu sheng, ze tou wei zhi zhong.*)
If clear yang, *i.e.,* power or strength, is not upborne to the head, the head will feel heavy.

All wilting, panting, and vomiting pertain to the upper [body].
(诸痿 喘呕，皆属于上 *Zhu wei chuan ou, jie shu yu shang.*)
According to this statement, all wilting, panting, and vomiting pertain to the upper. We would like to say that "upper" here means the upper burner. However, vomiting is a middle burner disease, although it manifests from the mouth which is in the upper burner. Wilting is often ascribed to the lungs, and panting is definitely primarily a lung disease. So wilting and panting not only pertain to the upper body but specifically to the lungs in the upper burner.

All reversal with constipation or diarrhea pertain to the lower [body]. (诸厥固泄，皆属于下 *Zhu jue gu xie, jie shu yu xia.*)
Constipation and diarrhea are ultimately intestinal diseases, and the intestines are located in the lower half of the body. Therefore, all constipation and diarrhea pertain to the lower body.

Detriment above reaches below. (上损及下 *Shang sun ji xia.*)
On the one hand, this can mean that any condition above may affect organs or body parts below. However, if we interpret "detriment" to mean damage resulting in vacuity, then it means that vacuity of an organ in the upper burner may eventually affect an organ or body part in the lower burner. For instance, lung yin vacuity can evolve into lung-kidney yin vacuity. Similarly, heart yin vacuity may evolve in heart-kidney yin vacuity.

Detriment below reaches above. (下损及上 *Xia sun ji shang.*)
Again, this can simply mean that a disease below can affect organs and tissues above, or it can specifically mean that vacuity below may result in simultaneous vacuity above. For instance, kidney vacuity may result in spleen vacuity, and spleen vacuity may result in either or both lung and heart vacuity.

Withering of fluids [may lead to] blood dryness. (津枯血燥。*Jin ku xue zao.*)
Because blood and fluids share a common source, withering or consumption of fluids may lead to concomitant blood dryness.

Fluid depletion [may lead to] blood stasis. (津亏血瘀。*Jin kui xue yu.*)
This statement is an extension of the previous statement. Because the blood and fluids share a common source, consumption of fluids may lead to blood dryness which leads to blood stasis.

Fat people [have] lots of wind stroke. (肥人多中风。*Fei ren duo zhong feng.*)

Fat in people leads to the interstices being [too] dense and lots of depression [and] stagnation. The qi and blood have difficulty flowing freely [and] uninhibitedly. Therefore, many die from stroke. (人肥则腠理致密而多郁滞，气血难以通利，故多卒中也。 *Ren fei ze cou li zhi mi er duo yu zhi, qi xue nan yi tong li, gu duo zu zhong ye.*)
These two statements both explain that fat people are prone to stroke and how such stroke occurs. Because of the presence of phlegm which hinders and obstructs the free flow of qi and blood, they easily develop qi stagnation and blood stasis. Therefore, many fat people die from stroke.

[If there is] enduring disease [in] a vacuous person with the stools not freely flowing, this is vacuity blockage. (久病人虚，大便不通者，是虚闭也。*Jiu bing ren xu, da bian bu tong zhe, shi xu bi ye.*)

[If] the stools are loose [and] thin, the urine is inhibited. (大便溏薄，小便不利。 *Da bian tang bo, xiao bian bu li.*)

[In] children, the liver commonly has a surplus, the spleen commonly is insufficient, the kidneys [are] commonly vacuous, [and] the heart [is] commonly replete. (小儿肝常有余，脾常不足，肾常虚，心常实。 *Xiao er gan chang you yu, pi chang bu zu, shen chang xu, xin chang shi.*)

This statement expresses the common pathological tendencies in infants and small children. In this case, the liver tends to be hot and hyperactive, while the spleen is vacuous and weak until approximately six years of age. At the same time, the kidneys are vacuous until puberty and not fully mature until the early 20s. Because heat from the liver and stomach tends to float up and accumulate in the heart, the heart often is replete with internally engendered heat evils. The heart may also be replete with phlegm confounding its orifices.

[When] the three qi of wind, cold, and dampness combine, they make impediment... [If] wind qi is overwhelming, it makes moving impediment; [if] cold qi is overwhelming it makes painful impediment; [if] damp qi is overwhelming, it makes fixed impediment. (风寒湿三气杂而至，合而为痹也... 其风气胜者为行痹，寒气胜者为痛痹，湿气胜者为着痹。 *Feng han shi san qi za er zhi, he er wei bi ye... qi feng qi sheng zhe wei xing bi, han qi sheng zhe wei tong bi, shi qi sheng zhe wei zhuo bi.*)

[In] bleeding conditions, [there is] qi exuberance [and] fire effulgence 8-9 [times] in 10. (血证气盛火旺者，十居八九。 *Xue zheng qi sheng huo wang zhe, shi ju ba jiu.*)

According to this statement, bleeding is most often caused by heat evils having entered the blood aspect causing the blood to move frenetically outside its vessels.

Spitting blood conditions pertain to repletion patterns 6-7 [times] in 10... [they] pertain to vacuity cold 1-2 [times] in 10. (吐血证，属实证者十居六七... 属虚寒者十中一二。 *Tu xue zheng, shu shi zheng zhe shi ju liu qi... shu xu han zhe shi zhong yi er.*)

Similarly, this statement says that most spitting of blood or hematemesis is due to repletion and only seldom due to cold. In this case, the repletion is typically heat.

Cold, summerheat, dryness, dampness, wind, fire, the six qi, all cause cough [in] humans. (寒暑燥湿风火六气，皆令人咳嗽。 *Han shu zao shi feng huo liu qi, jie ling ren ke sou.*)
The implication of this statement is that contraction of any of the six excesses may result in cough. In other words, cough is not just due to one evil.

The five viscera [and] six bowels [can] all cause cough [in] humans, not just the lungs. (五脏六腑皆令人咳，非独肺也。 *Wu zang liu fu jie ling ke, fei du fei ye.*)
Similarly, this statement says that cough is not just a lung disease but that it can be caused by another of the five viscera or six bowels. In other words, while the proximate location of cough is the lungs, its ultimate cause may be rooted in any other organ.

[If there is] enduring cough in humans, one, [there is] abiding vacuity, two, [there is] abiding phlegm. (久咳之人，一着虚，二着湿。 *Jiu ke zhi ren, yi zhuo xu, er zhuo shi.*)
According to this statement, there are two factors present in all chronic cough conditions—vacuity and phlegm.

Without vacuity, [there is] nothing to make dizziness. (无虚不作眩。 *Wu xu bu zuo xuan.*)
This statement implies that some sort of vacuity plays a role in all cases of dizziness.

Fetal toxins are the toxins of father [and] mother's lifegate/ministerial fire. (胎毒者，即父母命门相火之毒也。 *Tai du zhe, ji fu mu ming men xiang huo zhi du ye.*)
According to this statement, fetal toxins are a species of heat evils inherited from the parents due to inflammation of one or the other's life-gate/ministerial fire.

Vacuity is the cause of hundreds of diseases. (虚为百病之由。 *Xu wei bai bing zhi you.*)

This means that many, many diseases are due to one kind of vacuity or another.

[If] something exists internally, [it] must [have] form externally. (有诸内，必形诸外。 *You zhu nei, bi xing zhu wai.*)

This means that diseases on the inside of the body typically manifest signs and symptoms on the outside of the body.

Deprivation of essence [and] qi leads to vacuity. (精气夺则虚。 *Jing qi duo ze xu.*)

If essence and/or qi become vacuous and insufficient, then there is vacuity.

TREATMENT PRINCIPLES
(治则, *zhi ze*)

In Chinese medicine, the treatment principles or treatment methods (治法, *zhi fa*) are the bridge between the disease diagnosis and pattern discrimination on the one hand and the treatment plan on the other. In other words, they are the logical link between the two. The disease diagnosis and pattern discrimination are descriptions of what is going wrong in the patient's body. In particular, it is the pattern discrimination which states the disease mechanisms at work. The treatment principles are then the theoretic statement of what needs to be done in order to neutralize those disease mechanisms. They tell the practitioner what to do and in what order of preponderance (as reflected in the order of arrangement of the treatment principles). Knowing what, in theory, needs to be done, the practitioner then chooses the actual medicinals or acupoints which embody or implement those treatment principles. Thus the treatment principles are extremely important in the professional practice of standard Chinese medicine.

The superior doctor doctors the country, the mediocre doctor doctors people, [and] the inferior doctor doctors disease. (上医医国，中医医人，下医医病。*Shang yi yi guo, zhong yi yi ren, xia yi yi bing.*)

According to this statement, the highest form of medical practice is to treat the society as a whole. If the society and the environment are not healthy, how can those who live there be truly healthy? The next best level is to treat people. This means to treat the person as a whole, not just their disease. It means to take into account and attend to all their needs as much as is practicable. The lowest form of medicine is to treat disease as if it were separate from the person manifesting the disease. Such disease-based treatment often leads to heroic and short-sighted treatments which may cure the disease but kill the patient, or cure the symptoms but not get to the root of the disease.

Treat [or treating] on the basis of disease discrimination. (辨病论治 *Bian bing lun zhi.*)

This means predicating treatment on the patient's disease diagnosis. For instance, for migraine headache, do this. For multiple sclerosis, do that. In other words, everyone with the same disease gets the same treatment. Unlike some other systems of medicine, while standard professional Chinese medicine does use the patient's disease diagnosis to help erect the treatment plan, it is only a secondary factor.

Treat [or treating] on the basis of a pattern discrimination. (辨证论治 *Bian zheng lun zhi.*)

This means predicating treatment on the patient's personally presenting Chinese medical patterns. In standard professional Chinese medicine, treatment is primarily predicated on the patient's presenting patterns and only secondarily on their disease diagnosis. In fact, treating based on the pattern discrimination is the hallmark of traditional Chinese medicine. It is what makes Chinese medicine the safe and effective, holistic medicine it is. Treating based on each patient's presenting patterns allows the practitioner to individually tailor a treatment plan to that patient's specific needs.

Same disease, different treatments; different diseases, same treatments. (同病异治，异病同治 *Tong bing yi zhi, yi bing tong zhi.*)

This statement is a corollary of the preceding statement. It means that patients with the same disease diagnosis may receive entirely different treatments if their presenting patterns are different. Conversely, patients with different disease diagnoses may receive essentially the same treatments if their presenting patterns are the same.

To treat disease, seek its root. (治病求本 *Zhi bing qiu ben.*)

This means that practitioners of Chinese medicine should not just palliate symptoms. Instead, they should seek the root causes and mechanisms of each patient's disease and then address those in order to eradicate the disease in its entirety.

Treat [when] there is no disease. (治未病 *Zhi wei bing.*)

The superior doctor treats [when] there is no disease. (上工治未病 *Shang gong zhi wei bing.*)

The superior worker treats [when there is] no disease. The mediocre worker treats [when there is] already disease. (上工治未病，中工治已病者。*Shang gong zhi wei bing, zhong gong zhi yi bing zhe.*)

The superior doctor doctors [when there is] no disease, the mediocre doctor doctors [when one is] on the point of [being] diseased, [and] the inferior doctor doctors [when there is] already disease. (上医医未病，中医医欲病，下医医已病. *Shang yi yi wei bing, zhong yi yi yu bing, xia yi yi yi bing.*)

According to these statements, the superior doctor should prevent disease from arising, not just seek to eliminate it after it has taken hold. It is treatment based on pattern discrimination that allows the Chinese medical practitioner to do this. Everyone exhibits some pattern of disharmony even though they may not be diagnosed as suffering from a particular disease. By addressing these constitutional or habitual patterns when they are still relatively mild, one can prevent them from becoming so severe as to eventually cause disease.

Early treatment prevents changes. (早治防变。*Zao zhi fang bian.*)

According to this statement, treatment early in the course of a disease prevents the disease from changing and getting worse.

Act in accordance with seasonal, geographic, and personal factors. (因时因地因人制宜 *Yin shi yin di yin ren zhi yi.*)

This statement is also an expression of the holism of Chinese medicine. The practitioner should take into account the season of the year, the environment in which the patient lives, and the patient's personal diet, lifestyle, family, and work situations when both discriminating the patient's patterns and erecting a comprehensive treatment plan.

[In] acute [disorders], treat the tip [or branch]. (急则治标 *Ji ze zhi biao.*)

Literally, the word "acute" here means "urgent" or "very rapid." This statement means that it is OK to simply palliate severe symptoms in acute conditions. After these tip or branch symptoms are taken care of, then the practitioner has the space to address the deeper root causes and mechanisms. For instance, all forms of bleeding are considered emergency or acute conditions in Chinese medicine. Therefore, based on this treatment principle, it is ok to stop bleeding by any means necessary or at hand. However, once the bleeding has been stopped or brought under control, then one should attempt to discern the underlying cause of the bleeding and eliminate or remedy that.

[In] moderate [*i.e.* chronic conditions], treat the root. (缓则治本 *Huan ze zhi ben.*)

Literally, the word "moderate" here means "relaxed" or "slow." This statement means that, in conditions where time is not of primary importance, one should take the time to find the root causes and mechanisms of the patient's disease and then remedy those.

[If] the upper is diseased, treat the lower. (上病治下 *Shang bing zhi xia.*)

[If] the lower is diseased, treat the upper. (下病治上 *Xia bing zhi shang.*)

These two statements mostly apply to acupuncture and its related modalities. According to these statements, if there is a disease in the upper body, we may select acupoints on the lower body to treat it and *vice versa.*

[If] yang is diseased, treat yin. (阳病治阴 *Yang bing zhi yin.*)

[If] yin is diseased, treat yang. (阴病治阳 *Yin bing zhi yang.*)

These two statements are often used in acupuncture, but they may also be used in internal medicine. In terms of acupuncture, they mostly mean choosing points on the connected yang channel to treat the corresponding yin channel or organ and *vice versa*. In terms of internal medicine, if yang is hyperactive, we may supplement yin so that healthy, exuberant yin is able to control yang. On the other hand, if there are yin evils, such as dampness and cold, we may supplement yang in order to warm and transform the yin evils.

Repletion [is treated by] draining. (实则泻之 *Shi ze xie zhi.*)

Vacuity [is treated by] supplementation. (虚则补之 *Xu ze bu zhi.*)

In Chinese medicine, the conception of health and disease is based on the Confucian doctrine of the mean (中用, *zhong yong*) which is also sometimes referred to as the middle way. Accordingly, all disease in Chinese medicine is due to something being either too much, *i.e.*, replete, or too little, *i.e.*, vacuous. Therefore, draining repletions and supplementing vacuities are the two most basic treatment principles in Chinese medicine. All other treatment methods are subcategories or species of these two broad principles.

Heat [is treated with] cold. (热者寒之 *Re zhe han zhi.*)

Chinese medicine is a form of heteropathy. In an attempt to bring the patient back to a normal healthy balance or norm, the middle, the practitioner supplies an equal opposite stimulus. Therefore, heat is treated with cold or by cooling it.

Cold [is treated with] heat. (寒者热之 *Han zhe re zhi.*)

Likewise, cold is treated by heat or warming it.

Eliminate that which intrudes. (客者除之 *Ke zhe chu zhi.*)

This means to eliminate from the body any evil guest or intruding qi.

Straying [is treated by] moving. (逸者行之 *Yi zhe xing zhi.*)

If some righteous qi strays from its normal place in the body, it should be moved back to where it came from.

Lodging [is treated by] attacking. (留者攻之 *Liu zhe gong zhi.*)

Any evil qi which is lodged in the body should be attacked in order to remove or destroy it.

Dryness [is treated by] moistening. (燥者濡之 *Zao zhe ru zhi.*)
Signs and symptoms of dryness in the body should be treated by
engendering fluids in order to moisten that which is too dry.

Tension [is treated by] slackening. (急者缓之 *Ji zhe huan zhi.*)
Here, the word translated as "tension" is the same word translated
above as "acute" or "urgent," while the word "slackening" is the
same word translated above as "chronic." Here, tension refers to
cramping which should be relaxed, another meaning of the word
缓 (*huan*).

Dissipation [or scattering is treated by] contracting. (散者收之
San zhe shou zhi.)
That righteous qi which is dissipated or scattered should be
gathered together or "contracted."

Taxation [is treated by] warming. (劳者温之 *Lao zhe wen zhi.*)
Taxation means fatigue due to overwork. Here, it is said that taxation should be treated by warming. That is because taxation consumes and damages yang qi, thus leading to vacuity cold.

Hardness [should be] whittled away. (坚者削之 *Jian zhe xiao
zhi.*)
In Chinese medicine, hardness as a pathological descriptive is usually
associated with masses. In this case, such hard masses should be
whittled away.

Binding [is treated by] dissipation [or scattering]. (结者散之 *Jie
zhe san zhi.*)
Binding is another term that is often applied to lumps, masses, and
especially nodulations. According to this treatment, bindings should
be treated by dissipation or scattering.

Fall [is treated by] lifting. (下者举之 *Xia zhe ju zhi.*)
Here, "fall" refers to downward falling of the central or clear qi.
This results in symptoms of prolapse, such as a prolapsed rectum,
uterus, or bladder. In that case, what has fallen should be treated by
lifting or raising.

High [rising is treated by] repressing. (高者抑之 *Gao zhe yi zhi.*)

This means that what has pathologically counterflowed upward should be repressed.

Fright [is treated by] calming [or leveling]. (惊者平之 *Jing zhe ping zhi.*)

In Chinese medicine, the word 平 (*ping*) always has a spatial connotation. The character describes the flat top of a table. It means to calm but also to make level. In this case, fright which has caused the qi to flow chaotically should be calmed but also leveled.

The mild [is treated by] counterflow [*i.e.*, going against]. (微者逆之 *Wei zhe ni zhi.*)

This means that mild conditions should be treated heteropathically, warming cold, cooling warmth, moistening dryness, etc.

The severe [is treated by] following. (甚者从之 *Shen zhe cong zhi.*)

This means that sometimes very severe conditions result in paradoxical presentations, such as false heat when the patient is really cold or false cold when the patient is really hot. In that case one might warm a false heat condition or cool a false cold condition. These would be examples of "following" treatment in the case of severe conditions presenting paradoxically.

[If] the form is insufficient, warm with qi. (形不足者，温之以气 *Xing bu zu zhe, wen zhi yi qi.*)

According to this statement, if the bodily substance is insufficient, one should warm (or supplement) the body using medicinals that supplement the qi.

[If] the essence is insufficient, supplement with flavor. (精不足者，补之以味 *Jing bu zu zhe, bu zhi yi wei.*)

However, if essence is insufficient, one should supplement the essence with medicinals that are high in flavor, that thick part of food which nourishes substance.

[If there is] profuse bleeding, do not sweat. (多血者无汗 *Duo xue zhe wu han.*)

Because blood and fluids share a common source, if there is
profuse bleeding, one does not want to lose any more fluids.
Therefore, one should not sweat the patient.

[If there is] profuse sweating, do not bleed. (多汗者无血 *Duo
han zhe wu xue.*)
Similarly, if there is profuse sweating, one does not want to lose any
more fluids. So one should not bleed the patient.

[If there is] heat, do not assail with heat. (热无犯热 *Re wu fan
re.*)

[If there is] cold, do not assail with cold. (寒无犯寒 *Han wu fan
han.*)
These are both straightforward statements of Chinese medicine's
therapeutic heteropathy. If the patient is hot, do not add more heat.
If the patient is cold, do not add more cold. This would only be
repleting repletion, *i.e.*, making a repletion even more replete.

Use heat to treat cold. (以热治寒。*Yi re zhi han.*)

Use cold to treat heat. (以寒治热。*Yi han zhi re.*)

**Supplement that which [is] insufficient; drain that which has a
surplus.** (补其不足，泻其有余。*Bu qi bu zu, xie qi you yu.*)

**Vacuity patterns should be supplemented; repletion patterns
should be drained.** (虚证宜补，实证宜泻。*Xu zheng xuan bu,
shi zheng xuan xie.*)
These statements are all likewise straightforward expressions of
Chinese medicine's heteropathy. Use heat to treat cold and cold to
treat heat. Supplement that which is insufficient and drain that
which is replete.

**Repletion speaks of an evil qi repletion which must be drained.
Vacuity speaks of a righteous qi vacuity which must be
supplemented.** (实言邪气实，则当泻；虚言正气虚，则当
补。*Shi yan xie qi shi, ze dang xie; xu yan zheng qi xu, ze dang
bu.*)

This statement is similar to the above. However, it makes clear that all repletions are repletions of evil qi, while all vacuities are vacuities of righteous qi.

Protect the stomach qi. (保胃气。 *Bao wei qi.*)

Do not assail the stomach qi. (无犯胃气 *Wu fan wei qi.*)

Because the stomach qi (meaning the spleen and stomach qi) is the latter heaven root of the engenderment and transformation of qi and blood, practitioners should always take care not to damage the stomach qi by any treatment they may administer. If the stomach qi is damaged, then there is no source for the engenderment of the righteous qi in order to fight evils.

Depressed wood [is treated by] out-thrusting. (木郁达之 *Mu yu da zhi.*)

Out-thrusting means to thrust the qi stagnation associated with liver depression upward and outward. In internal medicine, this is accomplished by using windy-natured exterior-resolving medicinals, such as *Chai Hu* (Radix Bupleuri).

Depressed fire [is treated by] effusion. (火郁发之 *Huo yu fa zhi.*)

Similarly, depressed fire should also be effused or emitted using acrid, windy-natured medicinals.

Depressed metal [is treated by] discharge. (金郁泄之 *Jin yu xie zhi.*)

Evils depressed within the lungs should be discharged or drained from the lungs.

Depressed earth [is treated by] despoilation. (土郁夺之 *Tu yu duo zhi.*)

If the spleen or stomach is depressed, such as due to the presence of food stagnation, this should be treated by despoilation or abduction. Despoilation here means to seize and take something away, thus to forcibly disperse.

Depressed water [is treated by] conversion. (水郁折之 *Shui yu zhe zhi.*)

Literally, the word 折 (*zhe*) means to break or snap. However, it also means to turn back, change direction, or convert. Depressed water in this statement refers to accumulated dampness. In this case, it should be forcibly led away.

In vacuity, supplement the mother. (虚者补其母 *Xu zhe bu qi mu.*)

Vacuity leads to supplementing its mother. (虚则补其母。*Xu ze bu qi mu.*)

Repletion leads to draining its child. (实则泻其子。*Shi ze xie qi zi.*)

In repletion, drain the child. (实者泻其子 *Shi zhe xie qi zi.*)
These four statements are based on five phase theory. If the child viscus according to the engenderment cycle is vacuous, one should supplement its mother. For instance, to supplement the kidneys, one might supplement the lungs. Conversely, if the mother viscus is replete, one might drain that repletion by draining the child viscus. So in order to drain the spleen, one might drain the lungs. This theory is used mostly in acupuncture with the five transport points (五输穴, *wu shu xue*) of the 12 regular channels.

[For] blood repletions, diffuse [and] breach [them]. (血实者宣决之。*Xue shi zhe xuan jue zhi.*)
Blood repletions refer to blood stasis. In this case, one should attack and drain them, thus diffusing and breaching them.

To treat wind, first treat the blood. (治风，先治血。*Zhi feng, xian zhi xue.*)
Wind is nothing other than frenetically stirring qi, and blood is the mother of qi. Therefore, if one supplements the blood, the blood will then mother or root the qi, thus automatically treating the wind.

To treat the blood, first treat wind. (治血先治风。*Zhi xue xian zhi feng.*)
According to this statement, if there is bleeding due to blood heat, first treat wind. Treating wind here means to use windy-natured

medicinals to rectify the qi and resolve depression. Then the root of blood heat will be eliminated.

Treat wind [and] blood [at] the same [time]. (风血同治。 *Feng xue tong zhi.*)

This statement says to treat wind and blood at the same time. In fact, this is what we actually do most of the time in clinical practice.

[For] diseases of the bowels, [one] should free [their] flow. (腑病宣通。 *Fu bing xuan tong.*)

Freeing the flow of the stomach means to abduct and disperse food stagnation. Freeing the flow of the large intestine means to free the flow of the stools, and freeing the flow of the bladder means to disinhibit urination.

[If] evils have already entered the viscera, [one] should not sweat. (邪已入脏，汗之不宣。 *Xie yi ru zang, han zhi bu xuan.*)

Sweating is primarily a treatment method for evils lodged in the exterior. In that case, sweating is believed to out-thrust those evils from the defensive exterior. However, if evils have already penetrated to the viscera or the interior, then one should not sweat. In that case, sweating will not eliminate the evils and runs the risk of damaging the righteous.

[If one] wants to supplement yin, [one] must seek yin within yang so that yin obtains yang's upbearing and the source spring is not exhausted. (善补阴者，必于阳求阴，则阴得阳升而泉源不竭。 *Shan bu yin zhe, bi yu yang qiu yin, ze yin de yang sheng er quan yuan bu jie.*)

According to this statement, when supplementing yin, one should also use one or more yang-supplementing medicinals. This is because yin and yang are mutually rooted and yang transforms and engenders yin.

To regulate the menses, first address the liver. [Once] the liver is coursed, the menses are automatically regulated. (调经肝为先，疏肝经自调。 *Tiao jing gan wei xian, shu gan jing zi tiao.*)

According to this statement, liver depression and heat are the two main causes of most menstrual diseases. Therefore, treating the liver is typically necessary in the treatment of any menstrual disease.

Once liver depression is coursed and resolved or liver heat is clear and cooled, the menses will commonly go back to normal.

[For] detriment of the heart, regulate the luxuriant [or the constructive and] defensive. (损其心者，调其荣卫。*Sun qi xin zhe, tiao qi rong wei.*)

This means that, for damage of the heart resulting in especially spontaneous sweating, one must harmonize the constructive and defensive.

[For] detriment of the lungs, boost the qi. (损其肺者益其气。*Sun qi fei zhe yi qi qi.*)

This statement says to boost the qi in case of lung vacuity. In this statement, the word 益 (*yi*) does not just mean to supplement but also implies the upbearing of the clear qi from the spleen to the lungs. In other words, there is a spatial dimension to the word when used in Chinese medicine.

[If one] would be good at treating phlegm, do not treat phlegm, treat the qi. (善治痰者，不治痰而治气。*Shan zhi tan zhe, bu zhi tan er zhi qi.*)

Because the qi moves and transforms water fluids and phlegm is nothing other than congealed fluids, to treat phlegm well, one must typically rectify the qi (理气, *li qi*) as well as transform phlegm (化痰, *hua tan*).

[For] external rheum, treat the spleen; [for] internal rheum, treat the kidneys. (外饮治脾，内饮治肾。*Wai yin zhi pi, nei yin zhi shen.*)

According to this statement, for externally contracted dampness, treat the spleen, but for internally engendered dampness, treat the kidneys. However, this statement should not be taken as an absolute in contemporary Chinese medicine. It is merely a rough guide to be applied when relevant.

If [one] desires to free the flow, first [one] must fill. (若欲通之，必先充之。*Ruo yu tong zhi, bi xian chong zhi.*)

Since qi moves all the contents of the channels and vessels and blood nourishes and, therefore, enables the function of the channels and vessels, if there is lack of free flow associated with qi and/or blood vacuity, one must use qi and/or blood supplementing medicinals as well as qi and/or blood rectifying medicinals.

[If disease] is located in the skin, sweat and effuse [it]. (其在皮者，汗而发之。 *Qi zai pi zhe, han er fa zhi.*)

This statement means that if evils are located in the skin, one should treat them by sweating in order to effuse the evils from the body.

[In] spring [and] summer, nourish yang, [while in] fall [and] winter, nourish yin in order to address the root. (春夏养阳，秋冬养阴，以从其根。 *Chun xia yang yang, qiu dong yang yin, yi cong qi gen.*)

Spring and summer are the yang seasons of the year, while winter and fall are the yin seasons of the year according to yin-yang theory. According to this statement, one should nourish yang or yin in their corresponding seasons. In the case of spring and summer, these are seasons where people are more active and, therefore, use up more yang qi. So it makes sense to nourish yang in those seasons. Likewise, fall and winter are times of quiet recuperation and storage. Therefore, it is appropriate to nourish yin in these seasons so that one will have abundant stores of yin when the warm, yang seasons roll around again.

[For] disease [in] winter, treat [in] summer. (冬病夏治。 *Dong bing xia zhi.*)

According to this dictum, for diseases which recur every winter, one may attempt to treat them in the summer. For instance, it is common to treat wintertime panting and coughing or asthma during high summer with a course of direct moxibustion on the upper back.

[For] disease [in] summer, nourish [in] winter. (夏病冬养。 *Xia bing dong yang.*)

In this case, for diseases due to overconsumption of yin, blood, and fluids in summer leading to hyperactivity of yang, nourish and enrich yin, blood, and fluids in the winter.

First quiet [and there will be] no contraction of evils by earth. (先安未受邪之地。 *Xian an wei shou xie zhi di.*)

According to this statement, one should first quiet the spirit or mind to prevent contraction of evils by earth or the spleen. What this means is that one should quiet one's mind and prevent worry and anxiety from damaging the spleen. If the spleen is fortified (健, *jian*) and healthy (康, *kang*), the evils of earth, such as dampness, will not be able to harm the spleen.

External damage makes for having a surplus, [and that which] has a surplus [should be] drained. (伤其外为有余，有余者泻之。 *Shang qi wai wei you yu, you yu zhe xie zhi.*)
External damage means external contraction of evils, and all evil qi are species of repletion. Therefore, they should be drained.

Internal damage makes for insufficiency, [and that which is] insufficient [should be] supplemented. (伤其内为不足，不足者补之。 *Shang qi nei wei bu zu, bu zu zhe bu zhi.*)
Internal damage in this statement means internal damage of the five viscera. When the five viscera are diseased, in comparison to diseases in the exterior, they are more often due to vacuity, and vacuity should be supplemented.

If there is fullness and pain below the heart which is due to repletion, [one] must precipitate [this]. (按之心下满而痛者，此为实，当下之。 *An zhi xin xia man er tong zhe, ci wei shi, dang xia, zhi.*)
In this statement, "precipitate" specifically means to purge or precipitate the bowels, thus discharging replete evils from the stomach and intestines "below the heart."

[For] all diseases [which] do not heal, [one] must search within the spleen [and] stomach. (诸病不愈，必寻到脾胃之中。 *Zhu bing bu yu, bi xun dao pi wei zhi zhong.*)
The ability to fight off disease and heal is dependent on the righteous qi and the spleen and stomach are the root of the engenderment and transformation of the righteous qi. Therefore, non-healing diseases typically are complicated by at least some element of spleen qi vacuity.

The five viscera should be supplemented. (五脏宜补。 *Wu zang xuan bu.*)

The six bowels should be drained. (六腑宣泻。 *Liu fu xuan xie.*)
These two statements need to be read as a dichotomy. The first statement says that, in comparison to the bowels, the viscera should more often be supplemented than drained. Conversely, in comparison to the viscera, the bowels should more often be drained than supplemented. These two statements should not be taken as absolutes on their own.

The three yang [channels] should be needled; the three yin [channels] should be moxaed. (三阳宣针， 三阴宣灸。 *San yang xuan zhen, san yin xuan jiu.*)
Zhen jiu (针灸) means acupuncture *and* moxibustion, and each of these two modalities have their uses and indications. According to this statement, the three yang channels (of the hands and feet) should more often be needled as opposed to moxaed. The three yin channels (of the hands and feet), on the other hand, should more often be moxaed as opposed to needled. The implication in this statement is that needling is a more draining method and the three yang channels are more apt to suffer from repletion. Moxibustion is a more supplementing method and the three yin channels are more apt to suffer from vacuity.

[If] hyperactivity leads to calamity, continue to exert control. Controlling leads to engenderment [and] transformation. (亢则害，承乃制，制则生化。 *Kang ze hai, cheng nai zhi, zhi ze sheng hua.*)
According to this statement, if ascendant liver yang hyperactivity leads to calamity, such as stroke, continue to exert control, *i.e.*, continue to subdue yang, downbear counterflow, and clear heat. By doing this, the spleen's engenderment and transformation will eventually recuperate which will then aid the recuperation of the body. If one does not continue to drain the liver, the liver will continue to assail the spleen, thus preventing the engenderment and transformation of the qi and blood necessary to repair the body.

Bank earth to control water. (培土制水。 *Pei tu zhi shui.*)
This means to supplement the spleen to prevent the spilling over of water dampness.

Repress wood [and] support earth. (抑木扶土。 *Yi mu fu tu.*)

This means to course the liver and fortify the spleen in case of a liver-spleen disharmony.

Assist metal [and] level wood. (佐金平木。 *Zuo jin ping mu.*)

This means to supplement the lungs and drain the liver and downbear counterflow in the case of liver depression assailing the lungs.

Drain the south [and] supplement the north. (泻南补北。 *Xie nan bu bei.*)

This means to drain heart fire and supplement kidney water in the case of the heart and kidneys not interacting (心肾不交, *xin shen bu jiao*).

Use freeing the flow to treat [that which is] freely flowing. (以通治通。 *Yi tong zhi tong.*)

[For diseases] due to free flow, use freeing the flow. (通因通用。 *Tong yin tong yong.*)

Both of these statements are expressions of so-called contrary treatment. In this case, diseases characterized by excessive free flow are treated by freeing the flow. For instance, in the case of damp heat diarrhea, one may drain and discharge the intestines even though they are already seemingly draining and discharging.

Repress the strong [and] support the weak. (抑强扶弱。 *Yi qiang fu ruo.*)

This is another way of saying to drain that which is replete or overly strong and to supplement that which is weak or vacuous.

Support the righteous [and] dispel evils. (扶正祛邪。 *Fu zheng qu xie.*)

While this statement can mean to support or supplement the righteous qi and dispel evils in general, it is also a common principle for the treatment of cancer. In this case, Chinese medicine is used to support the patient's righteous qi, while surgery, radiation, and chemotherapy are used to dispel evils from the body.

Treat with food first; treat with medicine later. (食治为先，药治为后。 *Shi zhi wei xian, yao zhi wei hou*.)

[If] dietary therapy does not cure, then command [fate with] medicinals. (食疗不愈，然后命药。 *Shi liao bu yu, ran hou ming yao*.)

According to these statements, one should first treat with food and, only if this is not successful, secondarily treat with medicinals. In the second statement, the word 命 (*ming*) means both life or destiny as well as to command.

[If] the essence spirit [or psyche] is not taken into account [and] the mind not treated, disease cannot be cured. (精神不进，志意不治，病乃不愈。 *Jing shen bu jin, zhi yi bu zhi, bing nai bu yu*.)

According to this statement from the *Nei Jing (Inner Classic)*, if one does not take into account and treat the mind, one cannot cure the disease.

Those who would be good at doctoring, must first doctor the mind, and then later doctor the body. (善医者，必医其心。而后医其身。 *Shan yi zhe, bi yi qi xin, er hou yi qi shen*.)

This saying suggests that good doctors first treat the mind and only secondarily treat the patient's physical ailments.

Tranquilizing [or stilling] the spirit nourishes the qi. (静神以养气。 Jing shen yi yang qi.)

According to this statement, stilling or quieting the spirit nourishes the qi.

To quiet the spirit, one should be delighted [and] happy. (安神宜悦乐。 *An shen yi yue le*.)

This statement suggests that to quiet the spirit, one should help the patient be pleased or delighted and happy.

Stilling the heart contents the spirit. (静心怡神。 *Jing xin yi shen*.)

Treating the spirit is the root. (治神为本。 *Zhi shen wei ben*.)

Treating the spirit is the root of successful practice.

EVIL & RIGHTEOUS
(邪正， *xie zheng*)

In Chinese medicine, disease is seen as a battle between two forces—the righteous and the evils. The righteous qi is everything in the body which is healthy and normal. It includes the qi and blood, fluids and humors, essence and spirit. Evils include any externally contracted or internally engendered pathogens. If the righteous triumphs over evil, the person heals and recuperates. If evils overwhelm the righteous, disease worsens and may lead to death.

[In terms of] the qi in humans, [that which is] harmonious is the righteous qi, [that which is] not harmonious is evil qi. (气之在人，和则为正气，不和则为邪气。 *Qi zhi zai ren, he ze wei zheng qi, bu he ze wei xie qi.*)
This is the definition of righteous and evil qi in Chinese medicine.

If righteous qi exists internally, evil cannot offend. (正气存内，邪不可干 *Zheng qi cun nei, xie bu ke gan.*)

[If] the righteous qi [is] effulgent [and] exuberant, [it is] not easy to obtain disease. (正气旺盛，不易得病。 *Zheng qi wang sheng, bu yi de bing.*)

Any place where evils are, [the qi] is insufficient. (邪之所在，皆为不足。 *Xie zhi suo zai, jie wei bu zu.*)

[If] evils have occurred, the qi must be vacuous. (邪之所凑，其气必虚。 *Xie zhi suo cou, qi qi bi xu.*)
  All these statements say that, if there is sufficient righteous qi, evils cannot enter the body and disturb its function.

[If] the righteous qi is effulgent, even if there are strong evils, they are not able to affect [one. If they do] affect [one, the affection] must be light. Therefore, mostly [there is] no [or] the disease [is] easily healed. (正气旺者，虽有强邪，亦不能感，感亦必轻，故多无病病亦易愈。 *Zheng qi wang zhe, sui you qiang xie, yi bu neng gan, gan yi bi qing, gu duo wu bing, bing yi yi yu.*)
  This statement even goes on to say that, if the righteous qi is abundant and strong, even strong evil qi cannot enter the body or, if, by chance, such evils do enter the body, nevertheless, the disease will not be serious and will be easily cured.

The righteous qi attacks evils. (正气抗邪。 *Zheng qi kang xie.*)
  When the righteous qi becomes aware of the presence of evils in the body, it attacks those evils, trying to either force them back out of the body or destroy them.

The true [qi and] evils mutually struggle. (真邪相搏。 *Zhen xie xiang bo.*)
  Here, true qi is used as a synonym for the righteous qi.

The true [qi and] evils mutually attack. (真邪相攻。 *Zhen xie xiang gong.*)
  The relationship between righteous and evil qi is one of struggle or war. The righteous qi fights against the evil qi, and the evil qi fights against the righteous or true qi.

Evil qi [causes] detriment to the righteous. (邪气损正。 *Xie qi sun zheng.*)
  When the evil qi attacks the righteous, it attempts to damage and cause detriment to the righteous qi. Here, causing detriment means to cause the righteous qi to become vacuous, thus allowing the evil qi to grow and spread.

Exuberance of evil qi leads to repletion. (邪气盛则实 *Xie qi sheng ze shi.*)

Evil qi exuberance leads to repletion, essence [and] qi despoliation leads to vacuity. (邪气盛则实，精气夺则虚。*Xie qi sheng ze shi, jing qi duo ze xu.*)
> If evil qi is exuberant, then this is categorized as a repletion. If the essence and/or qi have been damaged or despoiled, this is categorized as vacuity.

[When] evil qi is exuberant, righteous qi becomes debilitated. (邪气盛者，正气衰也 *Xie qi sheng zhe, zheng qi shuai ye.*)

When evil collects, one's qi necessarily becomes vacuous. (邪之所凑，其气必虚 *Xie zhi sou cou, qi qi bi xu.*)
> Evil qi damages the righteous qi causing it to become less. Eventually, if the evil qi is not removed, the righteous qi will become vacuous.

If one does not have righteous qi to recover, evil qi will not retreat. (未有正气复而邪不退者 *Wei you zheng qi fu er xie bu tui zhe.*)

When righteous qi receives damage, evil qi begins to spread. (正气受伤，邪气始张 *Zheng qi shou shang, xie qi shi zhang.*)
> If the righteous qi is insufficient or damaged and becomes vacuous, this will allow the evil qi to spread through the body and become stronger and stronger.

If righteous qi is not exhausted, one's life cannot collapse. (未有正气竭而命不倾者 *Wei you zheng qi jie er ming bu qing zhe.*)
> As long as there is righteous qi left, the battle goes on and one will not die.

[If] the righteous [is] sufficient, evils [are] automatically removed. (正足邪自去。*Zheng zu xie zi qu.*)
> This means that sufficient righteous qi will be able to dispel or eliminate evils from the body.

[If] the righteous is exuberant, evils recede. (正盛邪退。 *Zheng sheng xie tui.*)

This means that, as the righteous becomes more and more exuberant, evils recede and retreat or abate.

[If] evils [have been] removed, the righteous [is] automatically quiet. (邪去正自安。 *Xie qu zheng zi an.*)

[If] evils [are] removed, the righteous [is] quiet. (邪去则正安。 *Xie qu ze zheng an.*)

These two statements then go on to say, once the evils have been removed from the body, the righteous qi will automatically return to its normal, healthy state.

BIBLIOGRAPHY

English sources & dictionaries:

A Practical Dictionary of Chinese Medicine, Nigel Wiseman & Feng Ye, Paradigm Publications, Brookline, MA, 1998

Basic Theory of Traditional Chinese Medicine, Vol. 1 & 2, Zhang En-qin, editor, Shanghai College of Chinese Medicine Publishing House, Shanghai, 1994

Chinese-English Terminology of Traditional Chinese Medicine, Shuai Xue-zhong, Hunan Science & Technology Publishing House, Changsha, 1983

English-Chinese; Chinese-English Dictionary of Chinese Medicine, Nigel Wiseman, Hunan Science & Technology Publishing House, Changsha, 1995

Matthew's Chinese-English Dictionary, Revised American Edition, R.H. Matthews, Harvard University Press, Cambridge, MA, 1993

The Pinyin Chinese-English Dictionary, Beijing Foreign Languages Institute, The Commerical Press, Hong Kong, 2000

Chinese sources:

黄帝内经导读 *(Huang Di Nei Jing Dao Du, Guided Readings in the Yellow Emperor's Inner Classic)*, Fu Wei-kang & Wu Ji-zhou, Ba Shu Publishing House, Chengdu, 1988

黄帝内经素问 *(Huang Di Nei Jing Su Wen, The Yellow Emperor's Internal Classic: Simple Questions)*, Xu Yan-chun, editor, Chinese Medicine Ancient Books Publishing House, Beijing, 1997

金匮要略 *(Essentials from the Golden Cabinet [or Coffer])*, Zhang Zhong-jing, edited by Yu Zhi-jian & Zhang Zhi-ji, Chinese Medicine Ancient Books Publishing House, Beijing, 1997

金书医学：张元素 *(Jin Shu Yi Xue: Zhang Yuan Su, Golden Books of Medicine: Zhang Yuan-su)*, Deng Hong-xin, Chinese National Chinese Medical Publishing House, Beijing, 2006

金元四大医学家名著集成 *(Jin Yuan Si Da Yi Xue Jia Ming Zhu Ji Cheng, A Compendium of Famous Books from the Four Great Medical Schools of the Jin-Yuan [Dynasties])*, Ye Chuan & Jian Yi, editors, Chinese National Chinese Medical Publishing House, Beijing, 1995

刘奉五妇科经验 *(Liu Feng Wu Fu Ke Jing Yan, Liu Feng-wu's Experiences in Gynecology)*, Liu Feng-wu, People's Medical Publishing House, Beijing, 1982

难经 *(Nan Jing, Classic of Difficulties)*, Qin Qi-ren, editor, Science & Technology Literary Book Publishing House, Beijing, 1996

秦伯未医文集 *(Qin Bo Wei Yi Wen Ji, A Collection of Qin Bo-wei's Medical Writings)*, Wu Da-zhen & Wang Feng, Hunan Science & Technology Publishing House, Changsha, 1983

伤寒论 *(Shang Han Lun, Treatise on Damage [Due to] Cold)*, Zhang Zhong-jing, edited by Li Pei-sheng, People's Medical Publishing House, Beijing, 1991

孙思邈养生长寿之秘 *(Sun Si Miao Yang Sheng Chang Shou Zi Mi, Sun Si-miao's Secrets for Nourishing Life & Longevity)*, Zhang Shi-ying, Shanxi Tourism Publishing House, 1997

万病回春 *(Wan Bing Hui Chu, Returning Spring to the Tens of Thousands of Diseases)*, Gong Ding-xian, Chinese National Chinese Medicine Publishing House, Beijing, 1998

血证论 *(Xue Zheng Lun, Treatise on Bleeding Disorders)*, Tang Zong-hai, People's Medical Publishing House, Beijing, 2005

医林改错 *(Yi Lin Gai Cuo, Correcting the Errors in the Forest of Medicine)*, Wang Qing-ren, Chinese National Chinese Medicine Publishing House, Beijing, 1995

中医基础理论图表解 *(Zhong Yi Ji Chu Li Lun, Chinese Medicine Basic Theory)*, Si Chang-chun, People's Army Medical Publishing House, Beijing, 2005

中医基础理论图表解 *(Zhong Yi Ji Chu Li Lun, Chinese Medicine Basic Theory)*, Wang Xin-hua, People's Medical Publishing House, Beijing, 2001

中医基础理论图表解 *(Zhong Yi Ji Chu Li Lun, Chinese Medicine Basic Theory)*, Yin Hui-he *et al.* Shanghai Science & Technology Publishing House, Shanghai, 1984

中医基础理论图表解 *(Zhong Yi Ji Chu Li Lun Tu Biao Jie, Diagrams & Explanations of Chinese Medicine Basic Theory)*, Zhou Xue-xing, People's Medical Publishing House, Beijing, 2000

中医基础理论应考必读 *(Zhong Yi Ji Chu Li Lun Ying Kao Bi Du, Necessary Readings for Examination in Chinese Medicine Basic Theory)*, Chen Rong & Zou Jin-sheng, Shanghai Chinese Medical University Publishing House, Shanghai, 2002

INTEGRATED PHARMACOLOGY: Combining Modern
Pharmacology with Chinese Medicine
by Dr. Greg Sperber with Bob Flaws
ISBN 1-891845-41-1
ISBN 978-0-936185-41-3

INTRODUCTION TO THE USE OF
PROCESSED CHINESE MEDICINALS
by Philippe Sionneau
ISBN 0-936185-62-7
ISBN 978-0-936185-62-0

KEEPING YOUR CHILD HEALTHY WITH
CHINESE MEDICINE
by Bob Flaws
ISBN 0-936185-71-6
ISBN 978-0-936185-71-2

THE LAKESIDE MASTER'S STUDY OF THE PULSE
by Li Shi-zhen, trans. by Bob Flaws
ISBN 1-891845-01-2
ISBN 978-1-891845-01-7

MANAGING MENOPAUSE NATURALLY WITH
CHINESE MEDICINE
by Honora Lee Wolfe
ISBN 0-936185-98-8
ISBN 978-0-936185-98-9

MASTER HUA'S CLASSIC OF THE
CENTRAL VISCERA
by Hua Tuo, trans. by Yang Shou-zhong
ISBN 0-936185-43-0
ISBN 978-0-936185-43-9

THE MEDICAL I CHING: Oracle of the
Healer Within
by Miki Shima
ISBN 0-936185-38-4
ISBN 978-0-936185-38-5

MENOPAIUSE & CHINESE MEDICINE
by Bob Flaws
ISBN 1-891845-40-3
ISBN 978-1-891845-40-6

MOXIBUSTION: The Power of Mugwort Fire
by Lorraine Wilcox
ISBN 1-891845-46-2
ISBN 978-1-891845-46-8

TEST PREP WORKBOOK FOR THE NCCAOM BIO-
MEDICINE MODULE: Exam Preparation & Study
Guide
by Zhong Bai-song
ISBN 1-891845-34-9
ISBN 978-1-891845-34-5

POINTS FOR PROFIT: The Essential Guide to
Practice Success for Acupuncturists 3rd Edition
by Honora Wolfe, Eric Strand & Marilyn Allen
ISBN 1-891845-25-X
ISBN 978-1-891845-25-3

PRINCIPLES OF CHINESE MEDICAL ANDROLOGY:
An Integrated Approach to Male Reproductive and
Urological Health by Bob Damone
ISBN 1-891845-45-4
ISBN 978-1-891845-45-1

PRINCE WEN HUI's COOK: Chinese Dietary Therapy
By Bob Flaws & Honora Wolfe
ISBN 0-912111-05-4
ISBN 978-0-912111-05-6

THE PULSE CLASSIC:
A Translation of the Mai Jing
by Wang Shu-he, trans. by Yang Shou-zhong
ISBN 0-936185-75-9
ISBN 978-0-936185-75-0

THE SECRET OF CHINESE PULSE DIAGNOSIS
by Bob Flaws
ISBN 0-936185-67-8
ISBN 978-0-936185-67-5

SECRET SHAOLIN FORMULAS for the Treatment of
External Injury
by De Chan, trans. by Zhang Ting-liang & Bob Flaws
ISBN 0-936185-08-2
ISBN 978-0-936185-08-8

STATEMENTS OF FACT IN TRADITIONAL
CHINESE MEDICINE   Revised & Expanded
by Bob Flaws
ISBN 0-936185-52-X
ISBN 978-0-936185-52-1

STICKING TO THE POINT 1:
A Rational Methodology for the Step by Step
Formulation & Administration of an Acupuncture
Treatment
by Bob Flaws
ISBN 0-936185-17-1
ISBN 978-0-936185-17-0

STICKING TO THE POINT 2:
A Study of Acupuncture & Moxibustion Formulas
and Strategies
by Bob Flaws
ISBN 0-936185-97-X
ISBN 978-0-936185-97-2

A STUDY OF DAOIST ACUPUNCTURE &
MOXIBUSTION
by Liu Zheng-cai
ISBN 1-891845-08-X
ISBN 978-1-891845-08-6

THE SUCCESSFUL CHINESE HERBALIST
by Bob Flaws and Honora Lee Wolfe
ISBN 1-891845-29-2
ISBN 978-1-891845-29-1

THE SYSTEMATIC CLASSIC OF ACUPUNCTURE
& MOXIBUSTION
A translation of the Jia Yi Jing
by Huang-fu Mi, trans. by Yang Shou-zhong &
Charles Chace
ISBN 0-936185-29-5
ISBN 978-0-936185-29-3

THE TAO OF HEALTHY EATING ACCORDING TO
CHINESE MEDICINE
by Bob Flaws
ISBN 0-936185-92-9
ISBN 978-0-936185-92-7

TEACH YOURSELF TO READ MODERN
MEDICAL CHINESE
by Bob Flaws
ISBN 0-936185-99-6
ISBN 978-0-936185-99-6

TEST PREP WORKBOOK FOR BASIC TCM THEORY
by Zhong Bai-song
ISBN 1-891845-43-8
ISBN 978-1-891845-43-7

TREATING PEDIATRIC BED-WETTING WITH
ACUPUNCTURE & CHINESE MEDICINE
by Robert Helmer
ISBN 1-891845-33-0
ISBN 978-1-891845-33-8

TREATISE on the SPLEEN & STOMACH: A
Translation and annotation of Li Dong-yuan's
Pi Wei Lun
by Bob Flaws
ISBN 0-936185-41-4
ISBN 978-0-936185-41-5

THE TREATMENT OF CARDIOVASCULAR
DISEASES WITH CHINESE MEDICINE
by Simon Becker, Bob Flaws &
Robert Casañas, MD
ISBN 1-891845-27-6
ISBN 978-1-891845-27-7

THE TREATMENT OF DIABETES MELLITUS WITH
CHINESE MEDICINE
by Bob Flaws, Lynn Kuchinski &
Robert Casañas, M.D.
ISBN 1-891845-21-7
ISBN 978-1-891845-21-5

THE TREATMENT OF DISEASE IN TCM, Vol. 1:
Diseases of the Head & Face, Including Mental &
Emotional Disorders
by Philippe Sionneau & Lü Gang
ISBN 0-936185-69-4
ISBN 978-0-936185-69-9

THE TREATMENT OF DISEASE IN TCM, Vol. II:
Diseases of the Eyes, Ears, Nose, & Throat
by Sionneau & Lü
ISBN 0-936185-73-2
ISBN 978-0-936185-73-6

THE TREATMENT OF DISEASE IN TCM, Vol. III:
Diseases of the Mouth, Lips, Tongue, Teeth & Gums
by Sionneau & Lü
ISBN 0-936185-79-1
ISBN 978-0-936185-79-8

THE TREATMENT OF DISEASE IN TCM, Vol IV:
Diseases of the Neck, Shoulders, Back, & Limbs
by Philippe Sionneau & Lü Gang
ISBN 0-936185-89-9
ISBN 978-0-936185-89-7

THE TREATMENT OF DISEASE IN TCM, Vol V:
Diseases of the Chest & Abdomen
by Philippe Sionneau & Lü Gang
ISBN 1-891845-02-0
ISBN 978-1-891845-02-4

THE TREATMENT OF DISEASE IN TCM, Vol VI:
Diseases of the Urogential System & Proctology
by Philippe Sionneau & Lü Gang
ISBN 1-891845-05-5
ISBN 978-1-891845-05-5

THE TREATMENT OF DISEASE IN TCM, Vol VII:
General Symptoms
by Philippe Sionneau & Lü Gang
ISBN 1-891845-14-4
ISBN 978-1-891845-14-7

THE TREATMENT OF EXTERNAL DISEASES
WITH ACUPUNCTURE & MOXIBUSTION
by Yan Cui-lan and Zhu Yun-long, trans. by Yang Shou-zhong
ISBN 0-936185-80-5
ISBN 978-0-936185-80-4

THE TREATMENT OF MODERN WESTERN
MEDICAL DISEASES WITH CHINESE MEDICINE
by Bob Flaws & Philippe Sionneau
ISBN 1-891845-20-9
ISBN 978-1-891845-20-8

UNDERSTANDING THE DIFFICULT PATIENT: A
Guide for Practitioners of Oriental Medicine
by Nancy Bilello, RN, L.ac.
ISBN 1-891845-32-2
ISBN 978-1-891845-32-1

YI LIN GAI CUO (Correcting the Errors in the Forest
of Medicine)
by Wang Qing-ren
ISBN 1-891845-39-X
ISBN 978-1-891845-39-0

70 ESSENTIAL CHINESE HERBAL FORMULAS
by Bob Flaws
ISBN 0-936185-59-7
ISBN 978-0-936185-59-0

160 ESSENTIAL CHINESE READY-MADE
MEDICINES
by Bob Flaws
ISBN 1-891945-12-8
ISBN 978-1-891945-12-3

630 QUESTIONS & ANSWERS ABOUT CHINESE
HERBAL MEDICINE:
A Workbook & Study Guide
by Bob Flaws
ISBN 1-891845-04-7
ISBN 978-1-891845-04-8

260 ESSENTIAL CHINESE MEDICINALS
by Bob Flaws
ISBN 1-891845-03-9
ISBN 978-1-891845-03-1

750 QUESTIONS & ANSWERS ABOUT
ACUPUNCTURE
Exam Preparation & Study Guide
by Fred Jennes
ISBN 1-891845-22-5
ISBN 978-1-891845-22-2